DOWN'S SYNDROME (MONGOLISM): RESEARCH, PREVENTION AND MANAGEMENT

Down's Syndrome (Mongolism): Research, Prevention and Management

Edited by

RICHARD KOCH, M.D.,

Children's Hospital of Los Angeles;
Professor of Pediatrics, University of Southern California (Los Angeles)

and

FELIX F. DE LA CRUZ, M.D.

Special Assistant for Pediatrics,
Mental Retardation Program,
National Institute of Child Health and Human Development,
National Institutes of Health

BRUNNER/MAZEL, *Publishers* New York

The work upon which this publication is based was performed pursuant to contract Number 229250 of the National Institute of Child Health and Human Development.

Published by
BRUNNER/MAZEL, INC.

64 University Place, New York, N.Y. 10003

Library of Congress Cataloging in Publication Data
Main entry under title:
Down's syndrome (mongolism).

Proceedings of a conference, held Oct. 29 and 30, 1973, at Anaheim, Calif., sponsored by the National Association for Retarded Citizens.
Includes bibliographies.
1. Mongolism—Congresses. I. Koch, Richard, 1921-ed. II. de la Cruz, Felix F., ed. III. National Association for Retarded Citizens.
[DNLM: 1. Mongolism. WM300 K76d]

RJ506.M6D68 616.8'58842 73-93839

ISBN 0-87630-093-X

PROCEEDINGS OF A CONFERENCE ON DOWN'S SYNDROME (MONGOLISM): RESEARCH, PREVENTION AND MANAGEMENT

Co-sponsored by

Parent Organizations for Down's Syndrome
National Association for Retarded Citizens

Supported by

Mental Retardation Branch of the National Institute of Child Health and Human Development
National Institutes of Health

Organized by

Childrens Hospital of Los Angeles

RICHARD KOCH, M.D., CONFERENCE CHAIRMAN
FELIX F. DE LA CRUZ, M.D. CO-CHAIRMAN
GEORGE JOHNSON, CO-CHAIRMAN

Preface

In the field of mental retardation, research and treatment for Down's Syndrome (Mongolism) have constantly moved forward. So that we might assess the strides made in recent years, a national conference, under the auspices of the National Association for Retarded Citizens (NARC), the Mental Retardation Branch of the National Institute of Child Health and Human Development (NICHD), and the Childrens Hospital of Los Angeles, was held on October 29 and 30, 1973 at Anaheim, California. This conference was attended by over 800 individuals from all over the United States, Canada, and Mexico. Included in the attendance were professionals, and members of various community agencies working with the retarded, public schools, etc. Most interesting was the fact that about 60 percent were parents of Down's Syndrome individuals.

The conference was sponsored by NARC, funded by NICHD, and organized by the Childrens Hospital of Los Angeles. Over 20 professionals and ten parents of Down's Syndrome children cooperated to put together an outstanding scientific conference.

The theme was Down's Syndrome (Mongolism): Research, Prevention, and Management. Plenary sessions focused on etiology, prevention, modality of treatment and current research efforts.

Drs. Richard Koch and Felix de la Cruz, together with Mr. George Johnson, chaired the meeting. Mrs. Jeannette Rockefeller, former member on the President's Committee on Mental Retardation, gave an enthusiastic Keynote Address. Her great concern for handicapped individuals and the great need to involve the federal government, as well as community agencies, with these needs were highlights of her topic.

The conference speakers explored the needs of Down's Syndrome individuals and the role that parents can play. There was agreement that infant stimulation programs provide wide interest and are a popular new concept; however, more research is needed to establish these programs as a new adjunct in the treatment for Down's Syndrome. No new medication, as yet, was of proven value.

While prevention of this syndrome is our desired goal, there was much disagreement as to how this was to be accomplished. The participation of parents was gratifying and served to stimulate discussion in a constructive manner.

Much credit is due Frances Durkin, Assistant to Richard Koch, M.D. on the Down's Syndrome Conference, for her dedication in making these conference proceedings available to you.

Richard Koch, M.D.
Felix de la Cruz, M.D.

Contents

Contributors

OMAR S. ALFI, M.D.—Division of Medical Genetics, Childrens Hospital of Los Angeles.

KATHRYN E. BARNARD, R.N., Ph.D.—Professor of Nursing, University of Washington, Seattle, Wash.

MARY COLEMAN, M.D.—Private practice, Washington, D.C.

PAT DEL MONICO, M.S.W.—Coordinator of Mental Retardation Services, Kennedy Child Study Center, Santa Monica, Calif.

GEORGE N. DONNELL, M.D.—Department of Pediatrics of the School of Medicine, University of Southern California, and the Divisions of Medical Genetics and Child Development of Childrens Hospital of Los Angeles.

ROBERT B. EDGERTON, Ph.D.—Neuropsychiatric Institute, Center for Health Sciences, University of California, Los Angeles.

JOAN ELL, M.S.W.—Chief Counselor, Regional Center for the Developmentally Disabled, Harbor General Hospital, Torrance, Calif.

KAROL FISHLER, Ph.D.—Associate Professor of Pediatrics (Psychology), University of Southern California, School of Medicine, and Clinical Psychologist, Regional Center for the Developmentally Disabled, Childrens Hospital of Los Angeles.

LAIRD W. HEAL, Ph.D.—Director of Research, National Association for Retarded Citizens.

MICHAEL M. KABACK, M.D.—The Division of Medical Genetics, Harbor General Hospital, and the Department of Pediatrics and Medicine, University of California at Los Angeles, School of Medicine.

RICHARD KOCH, M.D.—Director, Division of Child Development, Childrens Hospital of Los Angeles.

JAAKKO LEISTI, M.D.—Medical Genetics, Harbor General Hospital, Alberta, Faculty of Medicine, Edmonton, Alberta, Canada.

ERNEST E. McCOY, M.D.—Department of Pediatrics, University of Torrance, Calif.

FRANK J. MENOLASCINO, M.D.—Chairman, Research Advisory Committee, Senior Vice President, National Association for Retarded Citizens.

SIEGFRIED M. PUESCHEL, M.D., M.P.H.—The Developmental Evaluation Clinic, Children's Hospital Medical Center, Department of Pediatrics, Harvard Medical School, Boston, Mass.

MRS. JEANNETTE ROCKEFELLER—President's Committee on Mental Retardation, Washington, D.C.

MARTIN J. ROSENFELD, M. D.—Orange County Regional Center, Orange, Calif.

JO C. RUBLEE—Genetic Clinic, Childrens Hospital of Los Angeles.

ROGER G. SANGER, D.D.S.—Director of Dentistry, University Affiliated Project, Childrens Hospital of Los Angeles, and Assistant Professor of Pediatric Dentistry at the University of Southern California School of Dentistry, Los Angeles.

DAVID J. SEGAL—Department of Pediatrics, University of Alberta, Faculty of Medicine, Edmonton, Alberta, Canada.

SUE SEITZ, Ph.D.—Department of Communicative Disorders, University of Wisconsin, Madison.

JACK B. SHARE, Ph.D.—Assistant Professor, University of California at Los Angeles, Graduate School of Education.

KENNETH N. F. SHAW, Ph. D.—Division of Medical Genetics, Childrens Hospital of Los Angeles.

GEORGE F. SMITH, M.D.—Rush Medical School, Chicago, Ill.

ZENA A. STEIN, M.A., M.B., B. Ch.—Director, New York State Department of Mental Hygiene, Epidemiology of Mental Retardation Research Unit, and Professor of Public Health, Division of Epidemiology, Columbia University, New York.

KEN STRYNADKA—Department of Pediatrics, University of Alberta, Faculty of Medicine, Edmonton, Alberta, Canada.

FLOYD R. SWANSON—Chief, Personnel Staffing Branch, Office of Personnel Management, National Institutes of Health, Bethesda, Md.

JOSEF WARKANY, M.D.—Professor of Research Pediatrics, Children's Hospital Medical Center, Cincinnati, Ohio, and Department of Pediatrics, College of Medicine, University of Cincinnati.

PHILLIP WEISE, Ph.D.—Division of Child Development, Childrens Hospital of Los Angeles and the Department of Pediatrics, University of Southern California School of Medicine, Los Angeles.

ELIZABETH ZAUSMER, M.Ed., P.T.—Developmental Evaluation Clinic and Department of Physical Therapy, Children's Hospital Medical Center, Boston, Mass.

DOWN'S SYNDROME (MONGOLISM): RESEARCH, PREVENTION AND MANAGEMENT

1

Introduction

JEANNETTE ROCKEFELLER

I feel that I should make a small confession to you regarding my remarks today.

For more than 20 years I have been an active volunteer in various areas of the broad field of health. In what might be called "person-to-person" service, I have worked as a volunteer in wards and in hospital and clinic settings. I have served as a trained volunteer case worker and as a family counselor. For many civic committees and organized health agencies, I have served as an elected officer, as a board member, in program planning, in legislation, and inevitably, in fund raising. In the final analysis, raising money is undoubtedly the most important work that volunteers can do, for without funds, no service, research or treatment program can hope to survive.

In looking back over a lifetime of health service, I realize that there are few, if any, volunteer assignments that I have not been asked to undertake. In the process of carrying out these varying responsibilities, I have made speeches. When I lump together the many political speeches, health speeches, radio and television appearances, and formal papers that I have delivered, the number tends to astonish me.

But the simple truth of the matter, and the basis of my confession to you today, is that I really do not enjoy making speeches, nor do I consider myself a particularly effective or dynamic public orator. When I am invited to speak, I invariably ask myself: "Why on earth do they want me?" and "What can I say that will be significant, helpful or meaningful?" I am acutely aware that I am merely a concerned volunteer, facing an audience of professionals and involved, knowledgeable parents and volunteers who doubtless know far more about the topic of the meeting than I. Every time I accept an assignment to deliver an address, and particularly a keynote speech intended to set a note of inspiration for an important meeting like this, I realize that I must be extremely audacious or extremely foolhardy to agree.

As a mother of healthy, normal children whose heart goes out to those who have not shared my good fortune, I have often asked myself how I might have felt, or what I might have done, had one of my babies been a Down's Syndrome child. This is not an easy or pleasant situation to conceptualize. In visualizing my reactions to such a personal dilemma, I find myself asking questions that are probably familiar to many of you:

"What could have caused this retardation in my child?"
"Am I in some way to blame?"
"Did I fail to provide the proper nourishment during pregnancy?"
"Was it hereditary?"
"Will it be safe for me to have other children?"
"Why did this have to happen to me?"

Would that we could provide positive, absolute responses to these questions. We can answer some of them in part. We can give opinions based on medical and practical experience. But many searching, troublesome questions about the cause, the disposition, the treatment, and the prevention of retardation remain unanswered.

Assuredly we are now much further along in our understanding of retardation than we were when I first became involved in this critical health issue many years ago. One of the most important aspects of meetings of this kind is that they permit us to look both backward and forward, to measure progress we might have made and evaluate priorities for future action.

How far have we come? I remember clearly and painfully within the framework of my own lifetime when the retarded child, particularly the Down's Syndrome child, was a social stigma, a black mark on the immediate community. Who of my generation cannot recall personal knowledge of children concealed in the home or banished to some remote institution in obeisance to society's silent, cruel condemnation of the retarded child as a representation of some ill-defined parental failure, or the harsh punishment of a vengeful God? We can all be grateful that these medieval concepts are evaporating.

Although we have not yet conquered mental retardation as a serious worldwide health problem, nor yet developed truly effective methods for prevention, we can at least take resounding heart in the knowledge that social values and public attitudes are changing. No longer are mental illness and mental retardation unmentionable, unspeakable disorders. Today the average American accepts retardation openly, offers sympathy and understanding to the child and the parents, and supports our efforts to alleviate and, hopefully, to eradicate the problem.

Certainly many pockets of resistance and public ignorance remain. We still have a massive public education challenge facing us. But I submit that attitudes can change and have changed. When thousands upon thousands of average citizens respond willingly to impersonal newspaper and radio invitations to spend a day in New York's Central Park embracing, loving, playing with and caring for retarded children, I think progress in creating a better climate of public understanding is clearly being demonstrated.

But such heartening evidences of changing attitudes seem insignificant when we evaluate how much more needs to be done. Were the public climate of acceptance and understanding truly universal, we would have no more Willowbrooks, no more overcrowded and understaffed facilities, no drastic shortages of research and treatment funds. A truly informed and aroused public would demand better prenatal care, better treatment, better evaluation, better care, and more research. Given the irresistible impetus of widespread, insistent public support, we could make giant strides toward normalizing and enriching the lives of retarded citizens.

Perhaps it might not be inappropriate to pause for a moment to consider why mental illness and mental retardation have for so many centuries been the target of such intense, bitter social rejection. Why have masses of people, albeit ignorant and weaned on superstitions and misconceptions, been so vicious in their mistreatment of the retarded?

The reason may be found at our most elementary level of thinking. From the beginning of time, the human mind has been the most unfathomable, mysterious part of the body. Even today, we understand *how* the mind works, but not *why*. Learned scientists can explain the mechanics of nerves, reflex reactions and even emotion, but *why* these mechanics work remains an enigma. The average human being, intuitively aware that the mind is a complex, mysterious, baffling, highly sophisticated control center for his total body, cannot help but feel acutely uncomfortable when faced with a mind that does not work properly or function at the so-called norm. Perhaps the shock of seeing someone undergoing an epileptic seizure is intensified by the fearful realization that we are seeing a mind that—even temporarily—has gone completely out of control. I believe that it is far easier for the average person to accept physical handicaps because we make a subconscious assumption that the mental capability of the handicapped person is unimpaired. The failure, the malfunction, or the abnormality of a mind is generally unsettling because it represents the greatest threat to the human condition.

We must, therefore, not be too surprised to find the public a little slow to react to our fervent pleas for understanding and compassion for those with mental retardation. In truth, if these assumptions be true, the fairly recent progress made in lifting some of the barriers of society that have surrounded mental retardation is all the more impressive. That retardation is no longer a "dirty word" should inspire us to redouble our efforts to obtain better public understanding.

In this important area of better understanding, we must not overlook our own limitations. Those of us who work for this health cause, both professional and volunteer, who have not had personal experience with the problem, must become increasingly aware of the tremendously conflicting emotions inevitable for the parents of a Down's Syndrome child.

Parents who must accept the knowledge that their child is mongoloid often veer from defensiveness to bewilderment to aggression. Often the mother's concern and love for her child lead to unrealistic dreams. She fantasizes that her devotion, her care and her dedication will be magical ingredients that will transcend genetic factors, and her child will be "cured." When professional judgment affirms and reaffirms her child's condition, she may easily become overly sensitive or quick to take offense. We know that it is not uncommon for distraught parents to sometimes turn on the very professional who is seeking to give them compassion, sympathy and guidance. For the professional, these occasional situations are vexing and frustrating; however, to understand them, we need only to put ourselves in the parents' place. How would we feel if life had dealt us such a shattering blow? How would we cope with some of the monumental and soul-searing issues that the parents of the Down's Syndrome child must face?

These issues are many and serious. Let us look at some of them for a moment:

Will institutionalization be best for my child? Perhaps it will spare other siblings in the home from traumatic familial problems. Perhaps the concerned, trained, objective attention of professionals will be the better way to maximize the growth and development of the Down's Syndrome child.

But can any institution, no matter how good or how well run, substitute for the benefits of home environment and family love? Will removing the child from the home, even for the hoped-for advantages of better education and training, compensate for the personal and public censure of "banishment" inherent in taking this step?

Can the child in the home setting truly be approached with objectivity? When the child remains in the home, even with the wisest and most enlightened professional guidance, it is always difficult for the mother in her interactions with the child not to try and make up for his limitations by becoming overly involved in his total existence. For the mother dealing with the Down's Syndrome child, it is difficult, if not impossible, to avoid overcompensating in loving, providing, supervising, catering, pampering and looking after. Excessive care for the mentally retarded child is a common maternal problem, if for no other reason than the unavoidable subjectivity the mother has in dealing with the child—feelings mixed with natural disappointment, penance and guilt. These emotions are usually inevitable.

Long-range issues continue to confront the parents. They cannot help but worry about the Down's Syndrome child's future. Will he be able to provide for himself? Where and how will he live? Should he require a lifetime of supervision, who will provide it? Who will look after, care for, and love this child when they are gone? These are troubling, often heartbreaking questions, and we do not as yet have sufficient positive answers for them.

Certainly much hope lies in the new concepts of normalization. Steps are now being taken to provide halfway houses and community living resources for older retarded individuals. These steps are still few and hesitant, but they do promise alternatives to institutional life.

Normalization as a treatment and life-style concept tends to establish certain minimum and maximum goals. The older person usually can be taught to care for himself, to dress and feed himself, to use household equipment, to do some kind of work, and to function to individual capacity. Experience has already shown that most Down's Syndrome children attend public special education schools, and some can master typing, sewing, operation of certain manual equipment, musical instruments, and other types of ordinary activities. Few acquire academic success, but other goals can be established that are realistic and attainable. These goals are most likely to be attained when everyone concerned with the child—parents, teachers, counselors, physicians—work upon the normalization basis of treating the Down's Syndrome individual as a person who can accomplish, work, rejoice, suffer, feel pain and happiness, and most important of all, love. Every living creature, even a plant, flourishes with love; the Down's Syndrome child responds to affection and love and gives as much as he receives.

In answering the parents' questions about insuring long-term, humane, comprehensive care, we are unable to give many guarantees. Certainly it would be marvelous if we could honestly state that local, state and federal governments were truly sensitive to and dedicated to meeting the long-range needs of the retarded. We have had few positive indications that this is the case. Governmental programs have helped, but they rarely come anywhere close to providing adequate solutions. In recent times, the converse is increasingly true.

It is difficult and perhaps dangerous to make general statements about local, state and federal programs for the retarded, since these programs vary widely and many are more effective than others. However, even to the most unprofessional and modestly informed eye, recent inequities are glaringly apparent. At one time, governmental grants to subsidize private programs covered the cost of the program. The current trend is for provision of partial funding, with the expectation that corporate and private philanthropy should fund the balance. While this may be a commendable premise in theory, in practice we have little or no means whatever to guarantee that the private sector will assume its share of the cost. Without some means of requiring cooperation from industry and the public, too much is left to altruistic initiative and the community's share is never received. Thus, programs wither and die.

Revenue sharing is another theoretical premise that reads well but so far fails to operate satisfactorily when put into practice. Without allocation or ear-marking or designation, revenues shared at the state and local level tend to fall into the hands of those closest to the till, and health programs have never been known to compete effectively with such long established sacred community cows as roads, highways and buildings. Decentralization of federal funding may be a sound conceptual approach, but in practice the fair distribution of funds is difficult, if not impossible, and the threat of creating countless local pork barrels is all too apparent.

We cannot in this brief time together answer or even deal with the multitudinous, knotty problems inherent in the total problem of mental retardation. The spectrum is vast and the needs are complex and serious.

What we can do is to assess priorities, determine next steps, and rededicate our energies and our convictions toward ultimate success. Rome may not have been built in a day, but it was built and it survives. We may have no magic wand to wave away the enormous obstacles to be overcome in solving the problems of mental retardation, but we do recognize what many of these obstacles are and we can plan together how we might surmount them.

You who meet here to consider research, prevention and treatment of Down's Syndrome have many assets in your favor, not the least of which is a burning, unquenchable determination to do something and achieve something in ameliorating the problem. Your courage, your dedication and your will to provide are those intangible factors that make the difference between failure and success.

In closing, let us look at our many tasks in the light of poetic lines written by one of America's greatest men of letters—Carl Sandburg.

Lay me on an anvil, O God;
Beat me and hammer me into a crow-bar.
Then let me pry loose old, crumbling walls.
Let me lift and loosen old foundations.
Let this prayer of steel be answered,
So that I may be the instrument to clear away
The ugly past, and make way for the
Better and brighter tomorrow.

We can indeed hope for a better and brighter tomorrow, if we work together in common cause to find ways to better fulfill the lives of these needful, deserving children who cannot help themselves.

2

Etiology of Down's Syndrome

JOSEF WARKANY, M.D.

Etiology is the science of causation of events and in our special case I plan to discuss causes of the disorder which we call Down's Syndrome.

Knowledge of the causes that bring about diseases and health disorders is of extreme importance to those who try prevention, since removal of causal factors can eradicate a disease. Many diseases of children have disappeared during the last few decades. We could close some of our hospitals for contagious diseases and our tuberculosis sanatoria. And some of the nutritional diseases that we saw as young physicians are not seen any more by our young colleagues. How long did it take to achieve these triumphs of modern medicine? I should say at least 150 years and probably longer since some of the foundations of rational medicine were laid before the nineteenth century. Thousands and tens of thousands of investigations contributed to the rich harvest we have witnessed in recent times. Throughout these years patients had to be treated to alleviate their suffering and attempts were made to prevent their diseases, but claims of success were often short-lived, since the answers were not around the corner.

Let us now turn to the etiology of Down's Syndrome. The first significant step in research on this syndrome was made in 1866 by Langdon Down, a London physician (1). His short description of the disease picture is a classic; its explanation as a racial deviation is wrong. There have been additions to Down's remarkable observations but the disease picture has continued as a diagnostic entity under the name "mongolism." It was found subsequently that the disorder occurs in all ethnic groups and the term "Down's Syndrome" has often been used instead of "mongolism." Physicians dealing with mentally retarded patients saw these "mongoloid" children among offspring of the rich and the poor, the intelligent and the ignorant; they saw them in the country and the cities, in the mountains and the plains. Explanations of this puzzling disease picture were many and for 93 years thoughts about its causation were abundant.

In preparation for a conference sponsored by the National Association for Retarded Children (NARC) through its Scientific Advisory Board (SRAB), I reviewed in 1958 the theories proposed in the past to explain the etiologies of "mongolism."

The explanations were of different type and different value. Some were based on observation; others were based more on speculation. Some contained a trace of truth; others did not. Some were well defined while others were so general that it was impossible to prove or to disprove them. In general the theories reflected the thinking of the times (2).

I have tried to arrange the theories in groups and shall say a few words about their background. References are available (3).

1. *Reversion to a primitive racial type.*
2. *Reversion to the Orangutan.*

By 1866 seven years had passed since the publication of Charles Darwin's challenging book on the *Origin of Species*. The excitement of the learned world is reflected in Down's explanation of mongolism as a reversion to a primitive racial type which seemed "to furnish some arguments in favour of the unity of the human species." Less understandable is the fact that 58 years later a book was written in England which explained *The Mongol in our Midst* as a reversion to the Orangutan (4). This book, which was taken seriously by some, appeared in at least three editions.

It was soon noticed that the mothers of many mongoloid children were of advanced age. This observation led to various theories which related maternal characteristics and disease to the origin of the child's disorder (5):

3. *Exhaustion by many pregnancies*
4. *After long periods of sterility*
5. *Diseased uterine mucosa*
6. *Abnormal implantation of egg*
7. *Uterine retroflexion*
8. *Increased amniotic pressure*
9. *Hypothyroidism*
10. *Hyperthyroidism*
11. *Maternal infantilism*
12. *Inadequate transfer of vitamin A from mother to child*
13. *Maternal worries*
14. *Diseases and accidents in early pregnancy*
15. *Maternal genetic predisposition and precipitating environmental factors.*

The long list of these possible causes shows that no specific maternal anomaly could be held responsible. Advanced maternal age remains an etiologic factor but it acts in a more subtle way than anticipated by early investigators. Many of these explanations were misleading because they blamed adverse events during pregnancy for the disorder. They promised that good care afforded the mother during pregnancy could eradicate the disease, a belief that led to many disappointments. There were legal implications too when accidents during the sixth or seventh week of pregnancy were adjudged to be the cause of the anomaly and awards were paid as compensation for injuries which had nothing to do with the child's Down's Syndrome.

Sometimes abnormal general conditions of the father or mother were held responsible:

16. *Alcoholism*
17. *Syphilis*
18. *Tuberculosis*
19. *Psychopathic background*

Parental and familial diseases probably were merely guilty by association. They were so prevalent that many parents were affected, but, as mentioned before, no class or group was safe from the affliction described by Down.

Many authors attempted to explain Down's Syndrome by a chief disturbance located in the patient's organism.

20. *Imperfect fetal development*
21. *Thyroid deficiency*
22. *Thyroid overactivity*
23. *Pituitary deficiency*
24. *Adrenal deficiency*
25. *Thymus deficiency*
26. *Gonadal deficiency*
27. *Polyglandular deficiency*
28. *Deficiency of an undiscovered endocrine gland*
29. *Fetal hyperthyroidism*
30. *Blockage of an enzyme system by an inhibitor such as fluorine at an early stage of development*

These theories led to recommendations for various treatments. It was the time of discovery of endocrine factors which could in mysterious ways alter the physical and mental qualities of persons whose body fluids were influenced by changes of the ductless glands. By now we know that in the child with Down's Syndrome every body cell is abnormal and we cannot deny that the endocrine glands of the patients are abnormal. But no gland is solely responsible for the entire disorder and no hormonal substitution therapy has been found to be a cure. Again disappointments of the parents were understandable.

As cell biology progressed, suspicions were pronounced that early disturbances at the time of or at times before conception were at fault. These suggestions, though too general, are still to be considered awaiting specific clarifications.

31. *Injury to germ cell or zygote*
32. *Cytoplasmic changes*
33. *Overaged or immature eggs*

In contrast to the authors who explained Down's Syndrome by environmental accidents which affect the mother during pregnancy there were others who attributed it to earlier, preconceptional and genetic alterations. But heredity was not obvious in the majority of cases, as Down's Syndrome is essentially a sporadic disorder. Consequently some complicated explanations were resorted to:

34. *Dominant with reduced penetrance*
35. *Hereditary disease due to one main recessive and other modifying genes*
36. *Five pairs of recessive factors or two dominant and four pairs of recessive factors carried in as many different chromosomes*
37. *Germinal mutation with consideration of chromosomal changes*
38. *Combination of microsymptoms in sibs and other relatives*
39. *Germinal (chromosomal) mutation* (7, 8, 9)

The desire to force the syndrome into Mendelian rules resulted sometimes in rather grotesque explanations which were not accepted by medical investigators nor by interested lay persons. But the theories listed under 37 and 39 proved to be correct (6, 7, 8, 9). An ophthalmologist and two pediatricians thought that the best explanation for Down's Syndrome would be a change in the number of chromosomes or an alteration of gross structure; they came close to the right answer at times when the correct number of human chromosomes was still unknown. Their theories could not be proved without the cytogenetic knowledge of later years.

This was the confusing status in 1958 when we prepared the conference on the etiology of Down's Syndrome in Cincinnati, but the situation was changed by the time we actually met in 1959. By then it had been announced by Lejeune and co-workers (10) that in nine mongoloid children cells from tissue cultures showed 47 chromosomes instead of the normal 46. And it was shown that in most cases of Down's Syndrome trisomy 21 could be demonstrated (11). This discovery was a decisive step forward. Many of the old theories could be discarded, particularly those that explained the disorder on the basis of events weeks after conception. Other theories which had been vague and too general before, were now confirmed in a more specific way. The presence of extra chromosomal material in every cell of the patient with Down's Syndrome appeared to be the solution of the entire problem.

But the children with Down's Syndrome are still with us and many are still being born. In medicine the riddle of a disease is not completely solved until we learn how to prevent it. And we cannot prevent Down's Syndrome as yet. We know several mechanisms that lead to the disorder but do not know enough about the causes of nondisjunction, translocation and mosaicism (12, 13). The search for their determinants must continue.

I have presented this overview because it shows how much patience and detachment it takes to work on etiologies which must be recognized to achieve preventive measures and eradication of a disease. Even poliomyelitis, which has almost disappeared before our eyes during the last 15 years, has a history of investigation through more than a century (15). The outstanding achievements of those who perfected the preventive vaccines are known to you, but such successes do not come from nowhere. They are preceded by invisible medical research that contributes a step here and a step there until the goal is reached. The public celebrates the harvest, but pays little attention to ploughing, sowing and tending of the growing plant. It is understandable that the public is impatient until the final goal is achieved. They are inclined to listen to those who promise quick solutions and shortcuts. We cannot blame them for that. But the serious investigators cannot give in to premature claims; they have to be critical and appear as spoilsports who stand in the way of rapid success. Refutation of unjustified claims is a tedious job but it is a necessary, though thankless, form of research which must go on until Down's Syndrome is reduced to a rarity, like the other diseases which have disappeared in our lifetime.

REFERENCES

1. DOWN, J. L. H.: Observations on an ethnic classification of idiots. *Clin. Lect. Rep. Lond. Hosp.* 3:259-262, 1866.
2. WARKANY, J.: Etiology of mongolism. *J. Pediat.* 56:412-419, 1960.
3. WARKANY, J.: *Congenital Malformations. Notes and Comments.* Chicago: Year Book Medical Publishers, 1971.

4. CROOKSHANK, F. G.: *The Mongol in our Midst.* London: Kegan Paul, Trench and Trubner Ltd., 1924.
5. SHUTTLEWORTH, G. E.: Mongolian imbecility. *Brit. Med. J.* 2:661-665, 1909.
6. SNYDER, L. H.: *Medical Genetics.* Durham, N. C.: Duke University Press, 1941.
7. WAARDENBURG, P. J.: *Das menschliche Auge und seine Erbanlagen.* The Hague: Martinus Nijhoff, 1932.
8. BLEYER, A.: Indications that mongoloid imbecility is a gametic mutation of degressive type. *Am. J. Dis. Child.* 47:342-348, 1934.
9. FANCONI, G.: Die Mutationstheorie des Mongolismus. *Schweiz. Med. Wschr.* 69:81-86, 1939.
10. LEJEUNE, J., GAUTHIER, M., and TURPIN, R.: Étude des chromosomes somatiques de neuf enfants mongoliens. *C. R. Acad. Sci.* 248:1721-1722, 1959.
11. LEJEUNE, J., GAUTHIER, M., and TURPIN, R.: Les chromosomes humains en culture de tissus. *C. R. Acad. Sci.* 248:602-603, 1959.
12. PENROSE, L. S., and SMITH, G. F.: *Down's Anomaly.* Boston: Little, Brown and Company, 1966.
13. HAMERTON, J. L.: *Human Cytogenetics.* New York: Academic Press, 1971. 2 Vols.
14. PAUL, J. R.: *A History of Poliomyelitis.* New Haven: Yale Univ. Press, 1971.

3

Chromosomal Abnormalities

GEORGE N. DONNELL, M.D., OMAR S. ALFI, M.D.
JO C. RUBLEE, *and* RICHARD KOCH, M.D.

Dr. Warkany has presented a general perspective on Down's Syndrome, including a discussion of the various hypotheses proposed to explain the findings in patients with this disorder. The possibility of an association with a chromosomal defect was suggested by a number of workers (1, 2, 3). In 1959, Lejeune, Gauthier and Turpin demonstrated that the chromosome number in cultures of the skin fibroblasts from nine patients with Down's Syndrome was 47 rather than the usual 46 (4). The extra chromosome was a small, acrocentric chromosome which was morphologically similar to the other two pairs of G group chromosomes in the cell. It was tentatively identified as chromosome number 21 (5, 6). In almost all patients with the picture of clinical Down's Syndrome, there is extra genetic material in all or some body cells. This is either an extra chromosome 21 or a major portion of this chromosome translocated to another autosome.

The chromosomal abnormalities in Down's Syndrome can be classified as follows:

a. Trisomy 21
b. Translocations
   (1) D/G (21 to 13, 14 or 15)
   (2) G/G (21 to 21 or 22)
   (3) 21 to other autosomes
c. Isochromosome 21
d. Mosaicism
e. Double aneuploidy

This work was supported in part by the Department of Health, Education and Welfare, Maternal and Child Health Service Project 422, and United States Public Health Service Grant AM-04135 and AM-04837.

TABLE 1

Sources of Referral to Childrens Hospital of Los Angeles of Down's Syndrome Patients, 1963-1973

	No.	%
Regional Center/CDC	491	60.0
Hospital	147	17.9
Local (5 counties)	95	11.6
Other in State	25	3.0
Out of State	61	7.4
Out of Country	1	.1
	820	100.0

TABLE 2

Age of 630 Down's Syndrome Probands at Time of Referral for Cytogenetic Study

	No.	%
Ist Day	3	.5
Neonatal Period	77	12.2
2 Mos. - 1 Yr.	184	29.2
2 Yr. - 4 Yr.	138	21.9
5 Yr. - 9 Yr.	124	19.7
10 Yr. - 14 Yr.	45	7.1
15 Yr. +	59	9.4
	630	100.0

Examples of these chromosomal defects have been encountered in our own laboratory, and the following discussion is based on this experience.

We have received samples for cytogenetic study from more than 800 individuals with Down's Syndrome during the past ten years. The referral sources of these patients have extended beyond the limits of Southern California, with 7.5% of the patients from other states (Table 1). The background of the patients included various ethnic groups. The ages of the patients at the time of the cytogenetic study were available for 630. These varied from the first day of life to late adolescence. Approximately 41% were referred during the first year of life, including 0.5% on the day of birth, and 12% during

TABLE 3

Cytogenetic Findings in 991 Probands Referred as Down's Syndrome

Total	Down's	Apparently Normal	Others	% overdiagnosed
991	814	144	33	17.8

TABLE 4

Referral Diagnosis in 752 Probands Cytologically Diagnosed as Trisomy Down's Syndrome

Total	Down's	Others	% Missed
752	746	6	0.8

the first month (Table 2). The age of referral in the total sample is not a reflection of the age at which a clinical diagnosis was first made. A number of children were referred primarily for documentation and counseling.

Although the diagnosis of Down's Syndrome usually can be established correctly on clinical grounds alone, a cytogenetic study confirms the diagnosis and provides a basis for genetic counseling. Most of the patients studied in our laboratory had a referral diagnosis which proved to be correct. For 991 patients referred, a clinical diagnosis of Down's Syndrome was confirmed for 814. The remaining 177 (18%) had either some other chromosomal abnormality or normal chromosomes (Table 3). In the reverse sense, for the entire group of 752 cytologically diagnosed trisomy Down's patients, the clinical diagnosis, at the time of referral, was missed in only 0.8% (Table 4).

Among 820 Down's Syndrome patients studied there were 752 trisomies (91.7%), 40 translocations (4.9%), and 28 mosaics (3.4%) (Table 5).

TRISOMY 21

Our experience is consistent with the general observation that trisomy 21 is by far the most common form of Down's Syndrome (7,

TABLE 5

Cytogenetic Varieties of 820 Down's Probands

	Trisomy 21	D-G	G-G	Mosaics	Total
Male	394	15	7	15	431
Female	358	8	10	13	389
Total #	752	23	17	28	820
%	(91.71%)	(2.80%)	(2.07%)	(3.41%)	

8). The cells which can be examined have an extra small acrocentric chromosome with the identical morphologic characteristics of chromosome 21. These include later labeling upon autoradiography, satellites often present, and characteristic fluorescent staining along the long arms.

The mechanism for the occurrence of trisomy 21 is faulty chromosomal separation during the formation of an ovum and more rarely of a sperm (Figure 1). One fertilized cell would have 47 chromosomes, and would be trisomic for 21. The other, with 45 chromosomes and a single chromosome 21, usually does not survive. This also could occur in the zygote at the first division, or possibly later in the early development, with unequal distribution of chromosome 21 among the resulting cells. This is a rare event, and for practical

FIGURE 1

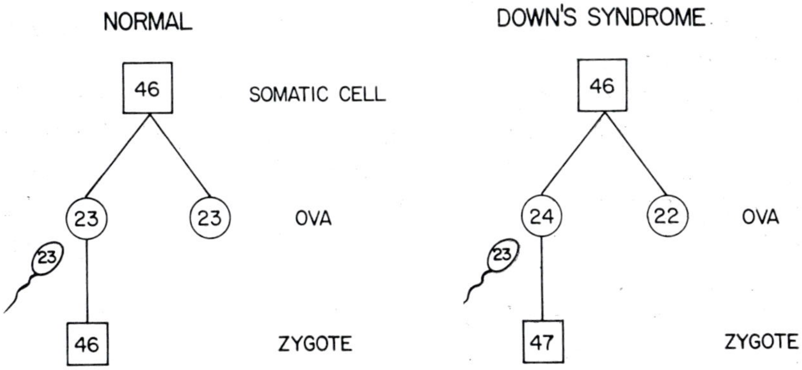

Mechanism for the occurrence of Trisomy 21.

purposes, the nondisjunction can be considered to occur in the gametes of one of the parents (usually the mother).

Among the hypotheses advanced to explain the causes of nondisjunction are aging of the ovum, familial predisposition, and environmental factors (9, 10, 11). Nondisjunction is usually ascribed to the mother, but a proportion of cases may be due to paternal nondisjunction.

TRANSLOCATION DOWN'S SYNDROME

Not all patients with Down's Syndrome have 47 chromosomes, but variations from the trisomy type comprise under ten percent of the Down's Syndrome population (12). Some patients have 46 chromosomes with a supernumerary chromosome 21 fused to another, usually a large or small acrocentric chromosome (D or G) (13). The translocation results from breaks which have taken place at or near the centromeres of the two chromosomes involved, followed by fusion at the site of the break (14). The most common translocation in Down's Syndrome is that from a chromosome 21 to one of the D group of chromosomes (chromosomes 13, 14 and 15) (Figure 2). Another less common form of translocation is one in which the extra chromosome 21 is attached to one of the G group (either 21 to 21 or 21 to 22).

Our series of 40 translocation Down's Syndrome patients included 23 D/G and 17 G/G.

With the introduction of banding techniques, a reliable way to differentiate between the carrier chromosomes in translocations became available (15,16). It was possible to study 12 of the 23 D/G translocations by these techniques. In nine of them a 21/14 translocation was identified, in three it was 21/15 and none proved to be 21/13. This is consistent with the observations of others that 21/14 is the most common of the D/G translocations and that 21/13 is rare (17,18).

Among 17 G/G translocations, eight were examined by banding techniques. There was one 21/22 translocation, and seven appeared to be 21/21 translocations. One of the latter turned out to be an

FIGURE 2

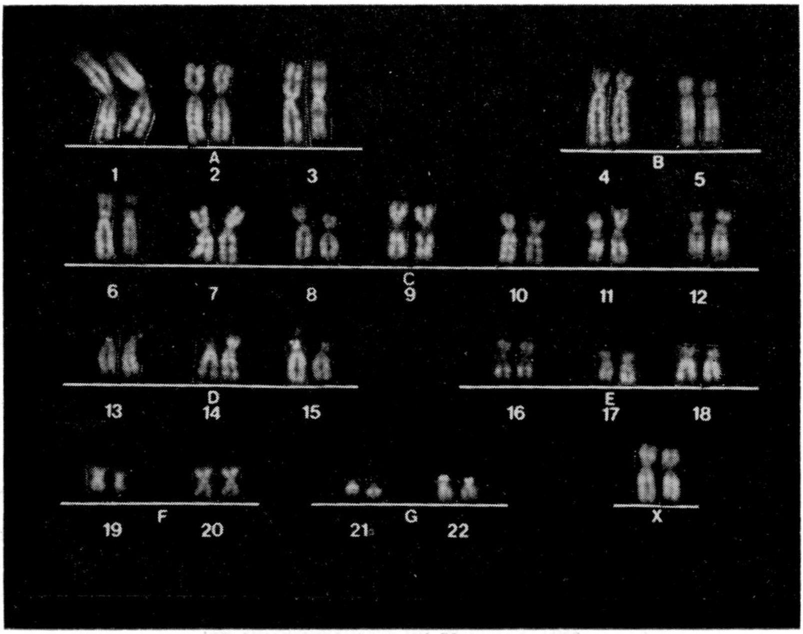

D/G translocation Down's Syndrome.

isochromosome for the long arm of 21. An isochromosome results from a chromosomal rearrangement which has taken place following a single break in the region of the centromere. Following the transverse break at the centromere, the two homologous half chromatids unite with each other and duplicate to form two new chromosomes, each of which is made up of identical arms. It is apparent that clinical Down's Syndrome due to an isochromosome for the long arm of chromosome 21 would be indistinguishable from that associated with a true 21/21 translocation. In the patient in question, three cell lines could be identified: a long arm 21 isochromosome, a short arm 21 isochromosome and a deletion of the short arm of chromosome 21 (Figure 3). These findings suggested an error in centromeric division resulting in the abnormal chromosome complement seen.

FIGURE 3

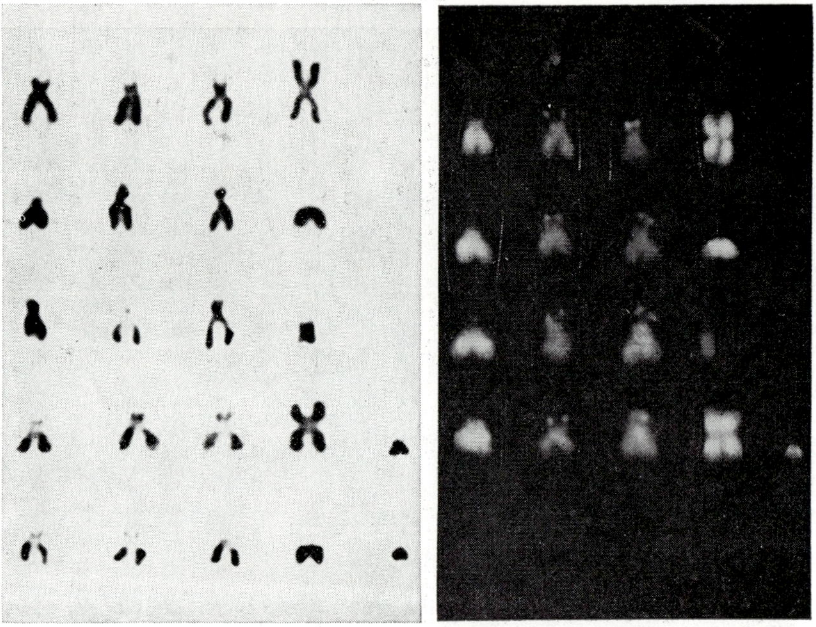

Karyotype of an isochromosome 21.

Although translocation Down's Syndrome accounts for only a small percentage of cases, such chromosomal defects are extremely important because either parent may be a balanced carrier of the translocation chromosome (Figure 4) with an increased risk of an affected child in a future pregnancy (19). The balanced carrier of a D/G translocation has 45 chromosomes. On karyotyping, a D group chromosome and a G group chromosome are missing, but are replaced by a chromosome resulting from the fusion of a chromosome 21 with one of the D group chromosomes. Translocation carriers are phenotypically normal because they have essentially the normal complement of genetic material.

Carriers of D/G translocations may have three types of offspring: chromosomally normal, phenotypically normal carriers, or translocation Down's Syndrome (20). A fourth possibility, 21 monosomy, is presumed to be lethal. The theoretical risk of having a translocation Down's offspring then is 1 in 3, but, from the practical standpoint,

FIGURE 4

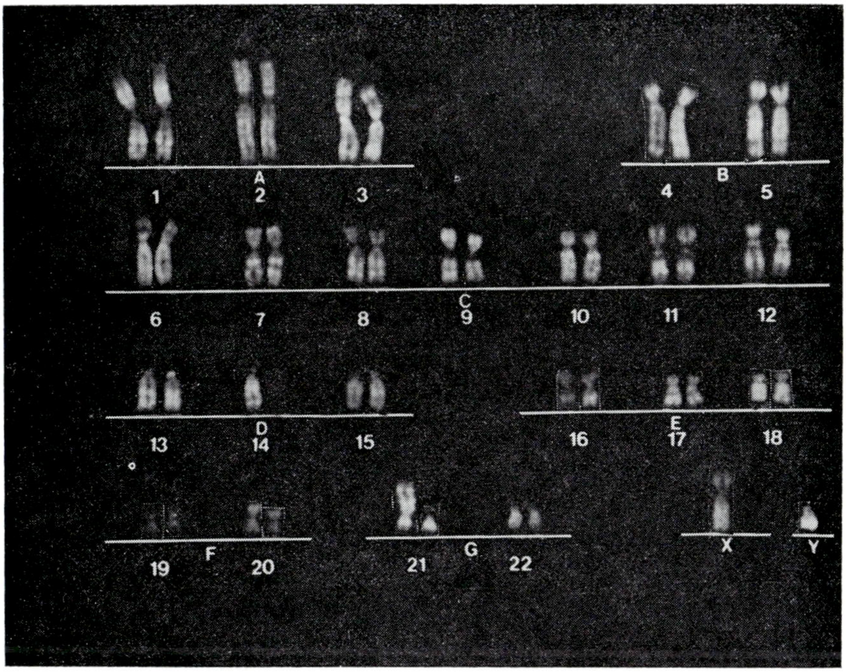

Karyotype of a D-G translocation carrier.

current estimates are 1 in 5 when the mother is the carrier, and 1 in 20 to 50 when the father is the carrier of the translocation chromosome (21). In D/G translocation, about one-third of the cases have a parent who is a balanced carrier, most often the mother (12, 22, 23). In reviewing our data on 23 D/G translocations, a carrier parent was identified in eight instances, a mother in seven and a father in one. In Figures 5 and 6 are presented pedigrees in which the transmission is illustrated.

No G/G translocation carrier parents were found in our group. It is important to distinguish between a 21/21 and a 21/22 translocation. A parent with a balanced 21/21 translocation cannot have a normal offspring. In contrast, carriers of balanced non-homologous translocations (21/22) can have offspring who may be either normal individuals or balanced translocation carriers, or have translocation Down's Syndrome (24).

FIGURE 5

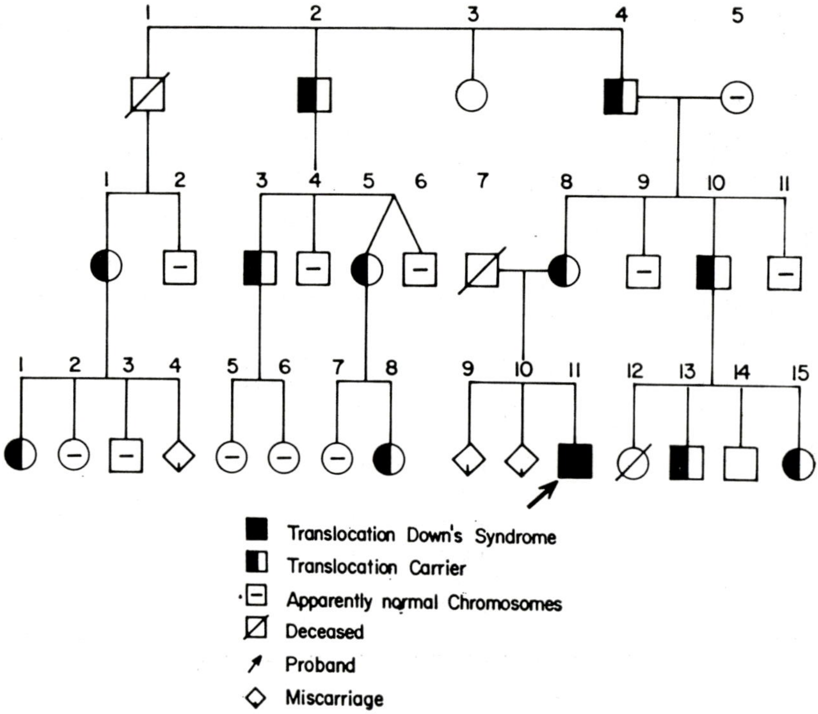

Pedigree demonstrating maternal transmission of a D-G (14-21) translocation.

G/G translocations, in contrast to D/G, seem to be more commonly transmitted through the father (25). Penrose found a significant increase in the paternal age in this group (26).

Although most of the translocations between acrocentric chromosomes presumably are centric fusions, the translocation occasionally occurs between the long arm of one chromosome 21 and the distal portion of the long arm of another 21 (tandem translocation) (27). One example is shown in Figure 7.

Translocations between a chromosome 21 and an autosome, other than in the D or G group, have been described, but these are very

FIGURE 6

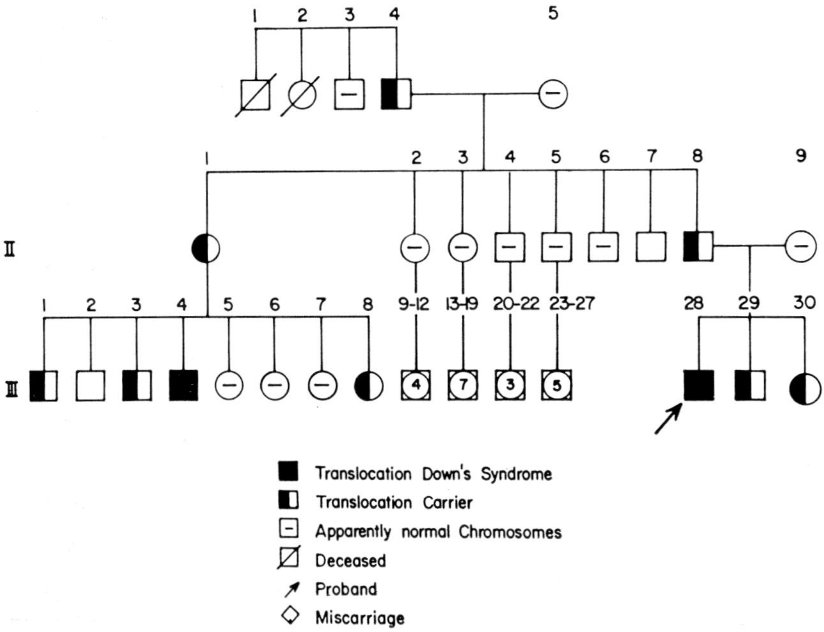

Pedigree demonstrating paternal transmission of a D-G (15-21) translocation.

rare (28). None has been found in our series. The implications are the same as for other autosomal anomalies following breakage and reunion.

MOSAICISM

In cytogenetics, mosaicism refers to chromosomal differences between cells present in an individual. The mosaic Down's Syndrome patient usually has two cell lines: one normal, and the other having one extra chromosome 21 (7, 8, 29). The phenotype of affected individuals may vary from virtually normal to typically affected. The clinical variability is thought to be related to the proportion of trisomic cells in the body as a whole or in a particular tissue (30,

FIGURE 7

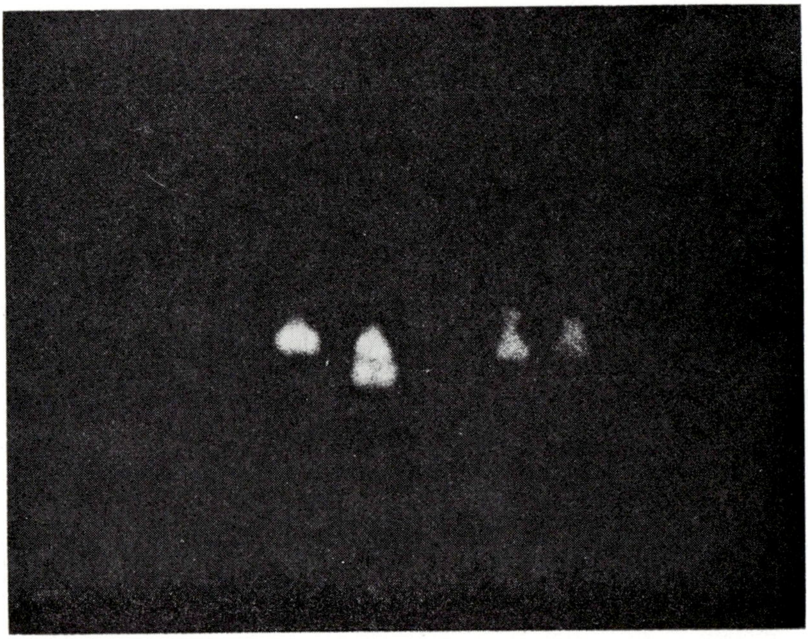

Tandem type 21-21 translocation.

31). There are individuals in the population who may have trisomic cells in one tissue, but who are phenotypically normal or almost so (32, 33).

If trisomic cells are confined to the ovary, they are difficult to identify. Penrose and Smith detected dermatoglyphic anomalies in about 10% of the mothers of Down's Syndrome children (34). They considered this to be evidence of mosaicism, involving the ovaries, which resulted in offspring with trisomic Down's Syndrome. Mosaicism also has been described in fathers of patients (35).

MULTIPLE ANEUPLOIDIES

Double trisomies have been described in patients with Down's Syndrome. In most instances these have been associated with triso-

FIGURE 8

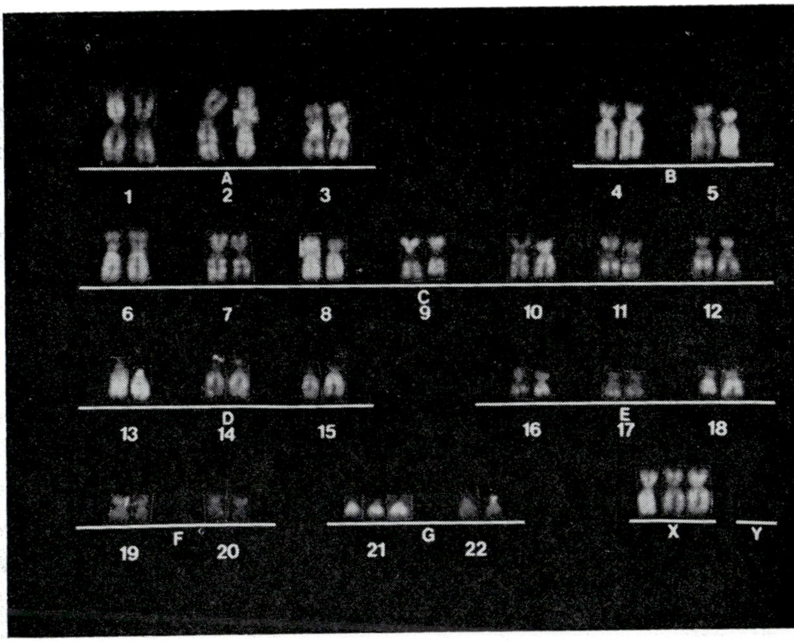

Karyotype of patient demonstrating double trisomy (21 and X).

mies of the X chromosomes (36). In our series, there are two patients with trisomy 21 and XXX and one individual who is trisomic both for 21 and 8 (Figures 8 and 9).

MATERNAL AGE EFFECT

Increasing maternal age is known to be associated with a greater likelihood of having a Down's Syndrome child (37, 38). The incidence of trisomy 21 goes up slowly until maternal age of 30, and increases sharply after age 35. However, the occurrence of translocation defects is not associated with maternal age. While the overall risk of giving birth to a baby with Down's Syndrome is approximately 1 in 700, the risk to a younger mother (19-20 years) is less than one in 2000 (39). At age 45 or over, the risk approximates

FIGURE 9

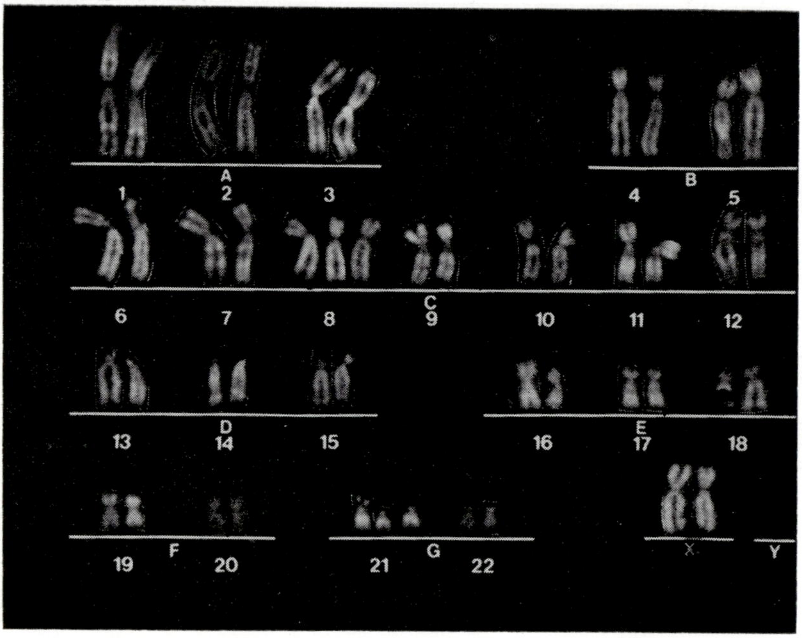

Karyotype of patient demonstrating double trisomy (21 and 8).

1 in 40. Possible causes of age-related non-disjunction in women include the aging process of ova, external environmental influences (irradiation, drugs, infection) and changes in sexual behavior (40). Data on maternal age at the time of birth of the Down's Syndrome child were available for 306 of the patients in our group. The mean maternal age was 31 years. The number of trisomy 21 Down's Syndrome births versus age of the mother at time of delivery is shown in Figure 10. The maximum number is for the 20-24 year maternal age interval, which corresponds to the peak of the fertility curve for the general population (41). Using the fertility curve as a basis, and assuming that our sample is representative of the Down's Syndrome population, the expected number of affected individuals per 1000 live births at various maternal ages was estimated. The resulting curve (Figure 10) corresponded closely to other studies, in that the

FIGURE 10

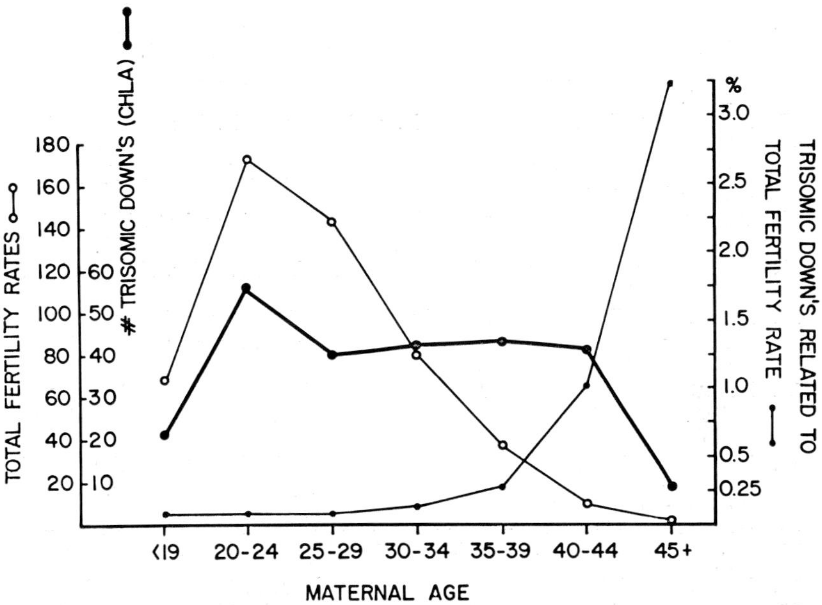

Occurrence of Down's Syndrome births at various maternal ages and the relationship of Down's Syndrome births to births in the general population.

risk of having a trisomic Down's child increased sharply after the maternal age of 35.

The need for cytogenetic studies in patients with Down's Syndrome for genetic counseling is evident. There are many questions yet to be answered, such as why additional genetic material produces an adverse effect and the possible consequence of loss of genetic material in the G/G and D/G translocations.

REFERENCES

1. BLEYER, A.: Indications that mongoloid idiocy is a gametic mutation of a digressive type. *Amer. J. Dis. Child.* 47:342, 1934.
2. PENROSE, L. S.: Maternal age, order of birth and developmental abnormalities. *J. Ment. Sci.* 85:1149, 1939.
3. WAARDENBURG, P. J.: Das menschliche Auge und seine Erbanlagen. *Bibliographia Genetica* 7:44, 1932.

4. LEJEUNE, J., GAUTHIER, M., and TURPIN, R.: Les choromosomes humains en culture de tissus. *C. R. Acad. Sci.* (Paris) 248:602, 1959.
5. BOOK, J. A., FRACCARO, M., and LINDSTEN, J.: Cytogenetical observations in mongolism. *Acta Paediat.* (Stockholm) 48:453, 1959.
6. LANCET. Leading Article. Complicating the chromosomal anomalies. 2:31, 1961.
7. HAMERTON, J. L., GIANNELLI, F. and POLANI, P. E.: Cytogenetics of Down's Syndrome (mongolism): I. Data on a consecutive series of patients referred for genetic counseling and diagnosis. *Cytogenetics* (Basel) 4:171, 1965.
8. CHITHAM, R. G. and MACIVER, E.: A cytogenetic and statistical survey of 105 cases of mongolism. *Ann. Hum. Genet.* 28:309, 1965.
9. PATAU, K.: The origin of chromosomal abnormalities. *Path. Biol.* 11: 1163, 1963.
10. MILLER, O. J., BREG, W. R., SCHMICKEL, R. D. and TRETTER, W.: A family with an XXXXY male, a leukaemia male and two 21-trisomic mongoloid females. *Lancet* 2:78, 1961.
11. FIALKOW, P. J., UCHIDA, I., HECHT, F. and MOTULSKY, A. G.: Increased frequency of thyroid autoantibodies in mothers of patients with Down's Syndrome. *Lancet* 2:868, 1965.
12. WRIGHT, S. W., DAY, R. W., MULLER, H. and WEINHOUSE, R.: The frequency of trisomy and translocation in Down's Syndrome. *J. Pediat.* 70:420, 1967.
13. POLANI, P. E., BRIGGS, J. H., FORD, C. E., CLARKE, C. M. and BERG, J. M.: A mongol child with 46 chromosomes. *Lancet* I:721, 1960.
14. ROBERTSON, W. R. S.: Chromosome studies I. *J. Morph.* 27:178, 1916.
15. CASPERSSON, T., ZECH, L., JOHANSSON, C., et al.: Identification of human chromosomes by DNA-binding fluorescent agents. *Chromosoma* 30:215-227, 1970.
16. SEABRIGHT, M.: Rapid banding technique for human chromosomes. *Lancet* 2:971-972, 1971.
17. HECHT, F. and KIMBERLING, W. J.:Patterns of D chromosome involvement in human (Dq Dq) and (Dq Gq) Robertsonian rearrangements. *Amer. J. Hum. Genet.* 23:361, 1971.
18. MIKKLESEN, M.: G group chromosomes, Birth Defects—Original Article Series, Part V, Phenotypic aspects of chromosomal aberrations. 50, May, 1969.
19. PENROSE, L. S., ELLIS, J. R., and DELHANTY, J. D. A.: Chromosomal translocations in mongolism and in normal relatives. *Lancet* 2:409, 1960.
20. HAMERTON, J. L. and STEINBERG, A. G.: Progeny of D/G translocation heterozygote in familial Down's syndrome. *Lancet* 1:1407, 1962.
21. ZELLWEGER, H.: Familial chromosomal aberrations, Part I. *Ann. Paediat.* (Basel) 206:317, 1966.
22. BREG, W. R., MILLER, O. J. and SCHMICKEL, R. D.: Chromosomal translocations in patients with mongolism and their normal relatives. *New Eng. J. Med.* 266:845, 1962.
23. CARTER, C. O., HAMERTON, J. L., POLANI, P. E., GUNLAP, A. and WELLER, S. D. V.: Chromosome translocation as a cause of familial mongolism. *Lancet* 2:678, 1960.
24. SHAW, M. W.: Familial mongolism. *Cytogenetics* 1:141, 1962.

25. FRACCARO, M., KAIJSER, K. and LINDSTEN, J.: Chromosomal abnormalities in father and mongol child. *Lancet* 1:724, 1960.
26. PENROSE, L. S.: Paternal age in mongolism. *Lancet* 1:1101, 1962.
27. ZELLWEGER, H., MIKAMO, K. and ABBO, G.: An unusual translocation in a case of mongolism. *J. Pediat.* 62:225, 1963.
28. KONTRAS, S. B., CURRIER, G. J., COOPER, R. F. and AMBUEL, J. P.: Maternal transmission of a 21/1 translocation associated with Down's Syndrome. *J. Pediat.* 69:635, 1966.
29. RICHARDS, B. W. and STEWART, A.: Mosaicism in a mongol. *Lancet* 1:275, 1962.
30. ZELLWEGER, H. and ABBO, G. N.: Chromosomal mosaicism and mongolism. *Lancet* 1:827, 1963.
31. VALENCIA, J. I., DE LOZZIO, C. B. and DE CORIAT, L. F.: Heterosomic mosaicism in a mongoloid child. *Lancet* 2:488, 1963.
32. HAMERTON, J. L., BRIGGS, S. M., GIANNELLI, F. and CARTER, C. O.: Chromosome studies in detection of parents with high risk of second child with Down's Syndrome. *Lancet* 2:788, 1961.
33. WEINSTEIN, E. D. and WARKANY, J.: Maternal mosaicism and Down's Syndrome (mongolism). *J. Pediat.* 63:599, 1963.
34. PENROSE, L. S. and SMITH, G. F.: *Down's Anomaly.* Little, Brown and Co., Boston, p. 118, 1966.
35. HSU, LILLIAN Y. F., GERTNER, M. LEITER, E. and HIRSCHHORN, K.: Paternal trisomy 21 mosaicism and Down's Syndrome. *The Amer. J. of Hum. Genet.* 23:592, 1971.
36. YUNIS, J. J., HOOK, E. B. and ALTER, M.: XXX 21-trisomy. *Lancet* 1:437, 1964.
37. CARTER, C. O. and MACCARTHY, D.: Incidence of mongolism and its diagnosis in the newborn. *Brit J. Soc. Med.* 5:83, 1951.
38. PENROSE, L. S.: Mongolism. *Brit. Med. Bull.* 17:184, 1961.
39. WARKANY, J.: Syndromes of chromosomal abnormalities. *Congenital Malformations (Notes and Comments).* Chicago: Year Book Medical Publishers, p. 313, 1971.
40. HIRSCHHORN, K.: Chromosomal abnormalities I: Autosomal defects. *Med. Genet.* Ed. by Victor McKusick and R. Clairborne, New York: Hospital Practice Publishing Co., p. 3, 1973.
41. U. S. Dept. H.E.W. Vital statistics of the United States, 1967.

4

Facial and Oral Manifestations of Down's Syndrome

ROGER G. SANGER, D.D.S.

For many years, before the advent of the numerous scientific achievements in medical research, the facial features of the human body were used as a primary diagnostic aid in the determination of the various genetic syndromes or disorders. More and more of these syndromes are being recognized, so that the clinician's diagnostic acumen is further challenged. No longer is the diagnosis of a genetic syndrome made solely on the basis of the configuration of the facial features or the characteristics of other organ systems, but rather by a combination of these physical manifestations and the various laboratory data now at the disposal of the clinician.

The face has been, and will continue to be, one of the most intriguing areas of the human body. The understanding of the embryogenesis of the human face and the manner in which various genetic and environmental factors can influence it is extremely important if our clinical progress is to keep pace with our laboratory and research progress. It is with these thoughts in mind that we must, at certain times, review our basic knowledge and understanding of a particular subject and ask ourselves new questions, so that we might better understand this process. The purpose of this report is to review our

Supported by Grant No. 914 of the Maternal and Child Health Service, Department of Health, Education and Welfare. Washington, D.C.

present knowledge of the influences that trisomy 21 exerts upon the embryogenesis of the human face.

THE FACE IN DOWN'S SYNDROME

The face comprises only one-third of the total mass volume of the skull and yet it is the most complex structure of the entire body, not only in its formation and development, but also in its anatomical architecture and configuration. The facial features of Down's Syndrome (trisomy 21) are numerous and, for this genetic disorder, have been considered to be pathognomonic (1, 2).

The accumulation of many parameters of craniofacial examinations has allowed us a rather vivid description of the clinical and radiographic features of the skull and the face, particularly in persons with Down's Syndrome. The skull can be noted to be small, brachycephalic, or rounded and often with an open metopic suture (3, 4). Thinness of the cranial bones has been reported, with almost an absence of diploe formation, as well as prominent convolutions or digital markings on the inner cortical laminae of the skull (5). This suggests that in Down's Syndrome, normal brain molding stress exists. It is more evident radiographically because of the increase in the digital markings and the thinness of the bones of the cranium without the diploe formation.

The forehead exhibits prominence; it has been described as bossing or bulging (1, 3). When measuring the height of convexity of the frontal bone, it can be shown that these individuals have a high degree of convexity, with the female showing more of this convexity than the male (5). This height of convexity is located more superiorly; however, maturation and development throughout adolescence and early adulthood tend to lower this height of convexity. The sinuses of the frontal area are often missing and when they are present, they are very minute in their formation. The supraorbital ridges may appear small because of this lack of development of the frontal sinuses (6, 7).

The nasal bridge has been described as flattened and broad, with the nose being both small and short (8). Absent, or malformed, nasal bones have been reported and this would account for the flattening of the nasal bridge (9). The length of the nasal bones, if they are present, is generally shorter than normal and the angle formed with the nasal complex more acute. The paranasal sinuses have a marked tendency to be underdeveloped, or missing entirely. The length of the anterior cranial base, as it is measured from the sella turcica to the nasal bones, is markedly less than normal in all ages. This anterior cranial base structure is also flatter than normal (5, 8, 9, 10).

Many persons with Down's Syndrome have the slanting, almond-shaped eyes with epicanthal folds and the oblique palpebral fissures. Strabismus is a common finding in over half of all these patients; however, it may be self-correcting later in life. Speckling of the iris or "Brushfield spots" can be seen in many patients. Increased occurrence of cataracts, along with a broad spectrum of other ocular manifestations, has been reported. Also quite common is ocular and bony orbital hypotelorism, which is probably a manifestation due to the lack of development of the frontal and nasal complex (3, 8).

The maxilla (upper jaw) is usually underdeveloped and hypoplastic. Cephalometric studies have shown (Figure 1) that the frontal process of the maxilla is underdeveloped in an anterior to posterior relationship, with the anterior nasal spine in a fairly normal position (5). This underdevelopment of the maxillary complex gives rise to the characteristic midface retrusion (posterior displacement) seen in these patients. With the underdevelopment of this region of the face, the inferior margins of the orbits may be positioned posteriorly with the anterior opening of the orbit facing more inferiorly. As the anterior opening of the orbits move anteriorly along with the maxillae, there appears to be a decrease in the angle of the anterior orbital opening. Thus, the obliquely situated orbits explain the oblique or mongolian slant of the eyes, along with the oblique palpebral fissures.

The underdevelopment of the frontal, nasal, and maxillary complex further accentuates the prominence of the forehead. As noted, however, the nasal and glabellar regions of the face have a forward growth vector, with the frontal area increasing in bony thickness. The supraorbital area, which may not be prominent due to the absence of the frontal sinuses, becomes longer and more elevated. The maxillary complex has more of a vertical or downward growth vector

FIGURE 1

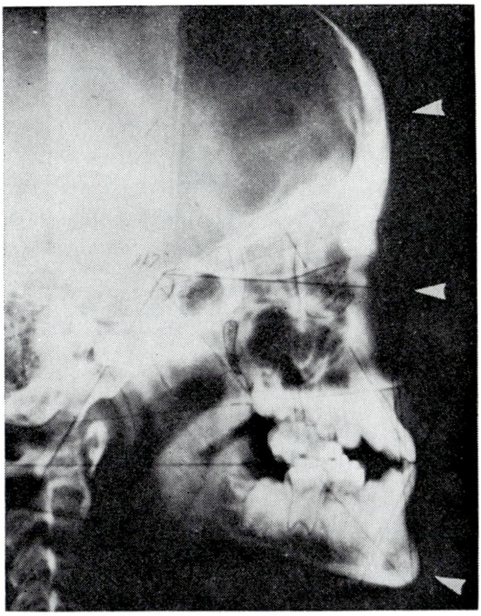

Cephaloradiograph of eight-year-old male with Down's Syndrome. The numbered lines are used to statistically compare the growth vectors of the craniofacial complex of this patient with normal controls. Note the frontal prominence (top arrow), the absence of a frontal sinus, the lack of forward development of the midface complex, the absence of the nasal bones (middle arrow), and the pseudoprognathic relationship of the mandible with the maxilla (botton arrow). Thinness of the cranium with an absence of diploe formation as well as prominent convolutions or digital markings can be seen in the frontal area.

than a horizontal or forward growth vector. With these growth changes there is much emphasis on the midface retrusion and the frontal prominence. However, even though this midface retrusion appears mild, it is further complicated by a normal growing mandible (lower jaw) which gives the characteristics pseudoprognathic appearance to the lower face, that is, the appearance that the lower jaw has exceeded its normal growth (5, 6, 7, 10).

Many parents and professionals outside of the dental profession have made inquiries about the lack of midface development. Generally these questions are in regard to the possible treatment of this maldevelopment. Oral and plastic surgical procedures have been alluded to in these inquiries. Hopefully, the previous discussion has implicated some of the complications in the easy solutions, or other surgical treatment approaches, for this midface maldevelopment. However, it should be emphasized further that the midface maldevelopment and its lack of sufficient forward growth are a direct result of the corresponding lack of growth of the anterior supporting base of the cranium, which supports the midface and its development. If this supporting structure is deficient or retarded also in its growth and development, then treatment of the midface, with its maldevelopment, is impractical.

The ears are generally malformed, and are often small in size and protrude at the helix. They appear to have an angular, overlapping helix and a prominent antihelix, with an absent or small lobe. The helix may also be absent. The positioning of the ears on the skull appears to be normal, although some authors have described the ears as positioned farther posteriorly on the skull than normal and abnormally rotated toward the posterior mastoid complex (3, 8).

THE ORAL CAVITY IN DOWN'S SYNDROME

The oral cavity is one of the complex organ systems of the human body. Its early embryogenesis and late maturation make it an excellent site for the scientist to investigate the genetic and prenatal and postnatal environmental insults.

The oral anomalies associated with Down's Syndrome are most easily recognized among the constellation of functional and physical disorders. These anomalies affect the jaws, the tongue, teeth, and the gingival and mucosal structures.

Thus it can be reemphasized that the maxillary complex lacks forward or frontal development and, therefore, occupies a retruded position in the facial complex, while the mandible exhibits normal growth and therefore, appears to be pseudoprognathic with respect to the underdevelopment of the maxillary and nasal complex.

The tongue in the individual with Down's Syndrome (Figure 2) has been described as being enlarged and fissured (11, 12). It often

FIGURE 2

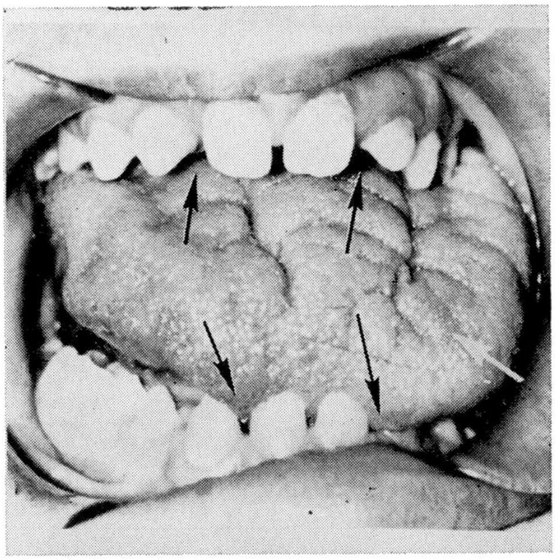

Photograph of the mouth and the tongue. Note the fissures of the tongue and its relative protruded position outside the mouth (white arrow). Note the lack of dental caries and the congenital absence of all the permanent lateral incisors (black arrows).

protrudes from the mouth. This is probably due to the minimal space allowed for the tongue to rest inside the oral cavity afforded by the pseudoprognathic position of the mandible and the underdevelopment of the maxillary and nasal complex. Consequently, the mandible is allowed to remain open and the tongue rests in the protruded position, outside the mouth, giving the illusion the tongue is grossly enlarged. Furthermore, the palatal vault height has been found to be normal, but with a narrowing and shortening of this vault. This deficiency in the palatal vault further limits the proper placement of the tongue in the mouth (13). The narrowing of the inferior and superior laryngeal apertures is caused by the high incidence of hyperplasia of the adenoids, laryngeal tonsils, and pharyngeal tonsils. Recently it has been reported that the open mouth and protruding tongue condition can be related to the functional need to provide adequate airway to compensate for the narrowing of the laryngeal apertures (14). This compensatory mechanism of breathing trans-

FIGURE 3

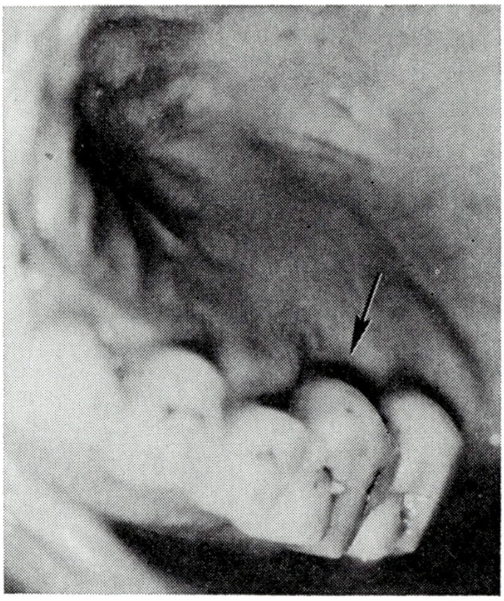

Photograph of maxillary right quadrant and palate. Note the lack of dental caries and the presence of severe periodontal disease adjacent to the crowns of the teeth (arrow). Palatal morphology is normal.

forms the person with Down's Syndrome into an obligatory mouth breather, which in turn dries the oral mucous membranes and the lips. The lips, however, are frequently subjected to a bathing of saliva from protrusion of the tongue and the resultant drooling. Inspiration and expiration of air over the lips dry the saliva, causing irritation and fissuring of the corners of the mouth.

The predisposition of the periodontium (gums) of Down's Syndrome individuals to disease has been one of the hallmarks of this genetic disorder (Figure 3). The severity of this disease is more exaggerated than usually seen clinically in other mentally retarded persons. The disease is suggestive of a Vincent's infection or periodontitis complex superimposed on an acute ulcerative gingivitis. Other mentally retarded individuals usually exhibit more of a chronic inflammatory disease (15, 16).

There can be marked alveolar bone degeneration, especially in the mandibular incisor region (17). With this periodontal disease and alveolar bone degeneration, the teeth can become progressively mobile in their bony sockets. They are often lost prematurely, due to the high incidence of abnormal occlusal function and the habit of bruxism (teeth grinding). Bruxism has been reported as being a frequent finding; in some cases it begins as early as two years of age. The traumatic and abnormal occlusal forces of bruxism can further precipitate periodontal destruction (18).

The formation of calculus, a known etiologic agent in periodontal disease, is neither common nor severe in these patients (16). Therefore, poor oral hygiene and the local factors of materia alba and calculus, proven etiological agents of disease of the periodontium, must not be considered to be the primary causes of this observed disease in Down's Syndrome (19). It can be postulated that these individuals have a greater susceptibility to periodontal disease, possibly due to an inborn error in the autoimmune mechanism in their systems, or possibly linked with alterations in the composition and metabolism of various products of the saliva, not found in other individuals.

The saliva has been the subject of numerous investigations, in view of the bizarre susceptibility of these individuals to periodontal disease, and also their low caries rate. It has been found that saliva, analyzed from the parotid gland, has a significant elevation in pH, as well as in sodium, calcium and bicarbonate ion concentration. The rate of flow, however, of parotid saliva is decreased when compared to normal salivary flow (19, 20, 21). The parotid saliva appears to have a higher concentration of uric acid, with no appreciable difference in total protein, creatinine, or amylase observed (21).

Electrolytes in the saliva of the submandibular gland were found to be within normal limits. However, the flow rate was again decreased. Thus, there appears to be an alteration in salivary gland metabolism in Down's Syndrome patients (19, 21).

The eruption of both the primary and permanent dentition of the child with Down's Syndrome is extremely variable and often retarded (8, 12, 16, 22, 23). This variability is far greater in these individuals than in the normal population (22). Generally, the first deciduous tooth enters the mouth between the twelfth and twentieth month, whereas in the normal population the first tooth appears between the fourth and sixth month. The primary, or deciduous, dentition may not be fully erupted before the fourth or fifth year (8, 19). The pattern of eruption is often quite variable. And this irregular pattern is often marked by the eruption of the deciduous molars prior to the eruption of the incisors (12, 22).

Anomalies of dentition, particularly those that affect tooth number, tooth morphology, tooth size, and tooth formation are present with varying degrees of concentration in all four of these categories of odontogenesis. The dental lamina of the first tooth germ starts its genesis around the thirty-third day in utero. The last developing tooth germ of the permanent dentition ceases its formation around the age of 16 to 18 years. It is easy for one to see that with this prolonged dental embryogenesis and maturation much individual tooth variation is highly probable and very likely to occur.

Anomalies of tooth number are often seen in the permanent dentition and are thought to occur about five times more frequently than in the normal population (8, 17, 24, 25, 26). One-fourth to one-half of all patients with Down's Syndrome are reported to have one or more congenitally missing teeth (19). The deciduous dentition also shares a high frequency of congenitally missing teeth, generally the lateral incisors (Figure 2) (6). In the permanent dentition this expression of abnormal tooth number is much broader and approaches the general population in the specific teeth that are most frequently missing congenitally. Yet, as previously mentioned, the individual with Down's Syndrome generally has five times more congenitally missing teeth than the general population. These congenitally missing teeth usually are the third molars, the second premolars, and the lateral incisors in descending rate of frequency (8, 16, 17, 18, 19, 25, 27).

Anomalies in tooth morphology are commonly seen (8, 12, 24, 25, 26, 27). Fusion of teeth in the deciduous dentition is frequently present. The maxillary lateral permanent incisor appears to be the tooth that expresses the most frequency of irregularity. The permanent premolars exhibit many irregularities of crown morphology and, in general, in most instances when an irregularity is present, its antimere has a similar irregularity (8, 25, 26).

Microdontia, or small teeth, have been observed in both the primary and the permanent dentition. The crowns of the teeth tend to be smaller than in the general population and the total length of the tooth, considering both the crown length and the root length, is much smaller. It has also been observed that the crowns of the teeth are asymmetrical in their formation. The females tend to exhibit more tooth-size variability than the males. The greatest dimorphism was noted in the mandibular canine (1, 8, 16, 18, 19, 26, 28).

The formation and calcification of the enamel portion of the teeth appear to be disturbed. This disturbance is thought to be a hypocalcification of the enamel due to the many developmental disturbances in fetal life that would insult amelogenesis (8, 19). These disturbances are seen less frequently in the general population. They can be detected microscopically in the ground sections of enamel of the primary dentition; they present themselves as prenatal enamel arrest lines (19).

Since infants with Down's Syndrome are frequently prone to infections that often require the administration of tetracycline antibiotics, the enamel of their teeth is often discolored. This discoloration is actually the intrinsic staining of the enamel by tetracycline, and does not represent an anomaly of formation attributed to Down's Syndrome.

The incidence of dental caries is extremely low (Figure 4) in comparison with other mentally retarded individuals and the general population (6, 16, 17, 18, 19, 24). This is very interesting from an etiological standpoint, since the known etiology of dental caries arises from poor oral hygiene and other dental abnormalities. The Down's Syndrome individual generally has very poor oral hygiene and a high frequency of dental anomalies, both of which would predispose the mouth to a high caries index. Low caries activity, furthermore, has been reported at a time when in the normal population there is a very high caries activity index (19). As was previously mentioned, much research is now being accomplished to determine if the altera-

FIGURE 4

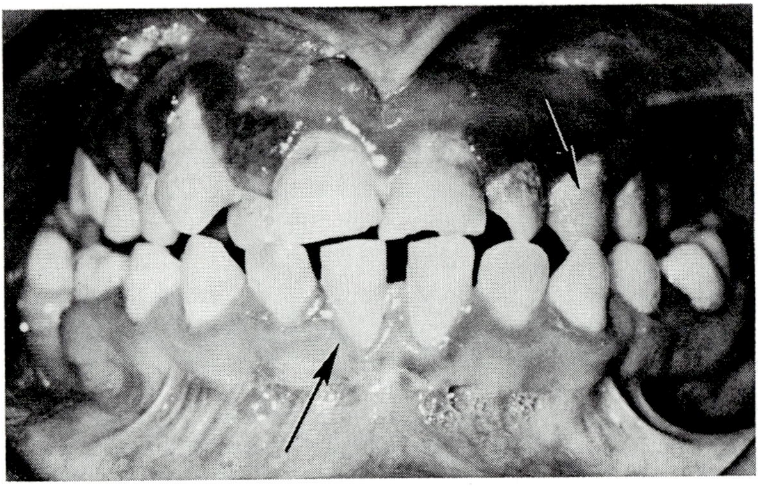

Photograph of mouth. Note the lack of dental caries in the presence of very poor oral hygiene and severe periodontal disease. Note the posterior crossbite with the mesiocclusion (top arrow). The lower incisors are mobile and spaces have developed due to alveolar bone degeneration and drifting of teeth (bottom arrow). The abrasions on the teeth are due to bruxism.

tion of the salivary metabolism is a possible postulate for this low caries activity.

Finally, with the aforementioned frequency of dental anomalies, it is not too uncommon that one would expect to find a high incidence of malocclusion in this same population. Malocclusion is present to some degree in almost all patients with Down's Syndrome. This malocclusion can be directly attributed to many of the characteristics of the face and dental anomalies (6, 12, 24, 29). And although all types of malocclusion have been reported as being present in this population, certain types do predominate. These include posterior crossbite, mandibular overjet, mesiocclusion or mandibular pseudoprognathism and anterior overbite (Figure 5), listed in descending order of frequency. All are related to the abnormalities that were described with the facial features. The underdevelopment of the maxillary and nasal complex is the prime contributory factor when assessing the etiology of the posterior crossbite and the mesiocclusion. The positioning of

FIGURE 5

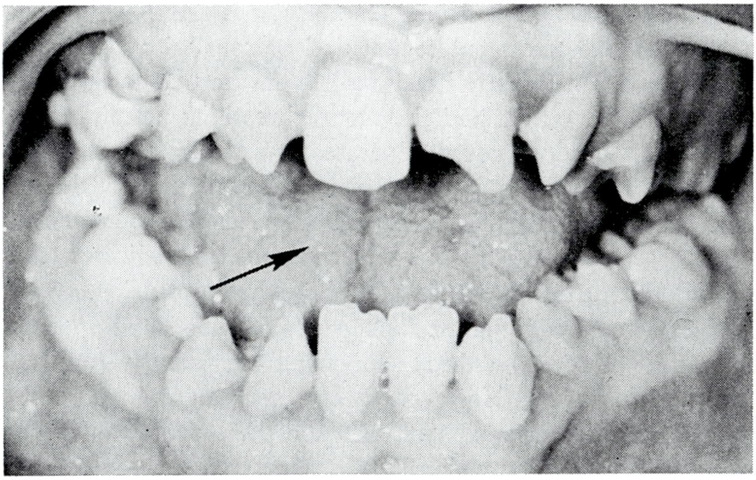

Photograph of the mouth. Note the anterior open bite (arrow) and the posterior crossbite. All four permanent lateral incisors are congenitally absent.

the tongue influences the formation of the anterior open bite. Irregularities in tooth size and formation, coupled with the maxillary basal bone discrepancy, contribute to the extreme crowding of the permanent and primary dentition in the upper jaw. However, the high frequency of congenitally missing teeth usually alleviates this problem of crowding since there are vacant spaces into which the crowded teeth may drift and stabilize.

Again, we receive many questions and inquiries regarding the development of the oral cavity. The tongue seems to be alluded to in most questions about this development. Solutions to the protrusion of the tongue have ranged from manipulation with various desensitizing devices to partial surgical resections. As mentioned previously, the tongue is generally not large, but rather normal in size and shape. It does protrude in some patients with Down's Syndrome due to the lack of midface and pharyngeal development. With this deficiency in the upper jaw and throat it becomes necessary to open the mouth and extend the tongue in order to breathe better. As this abnormal function continues, the nasal cavity suffers from disuse and becomes obstructed as the mucosa dries. Therefore, it is extremely important that early in the treatment regimen of persons with Down's Syndrome stimulation therapy be started to ensure that the tongue remains inside the mouth and the mouth breathing be minimized so the nasal cavity does not degenerate from disuse. And since the tonsils and adenoids in these patients are hyperplastic, these will definitely cause protrusion of the tongue. An examination and evaluation of these structures with possible treatment, if indicated, should precede any treatment regimen for this tongue protrusion.

Since Down's Syndrome persons generally have small upper jaws and palate, the teeth on these supporting bones suffer from many forms of malocclusion. However, there is generally a high incidence of missing teeth which compensates for the overcrowding that is usually present in these malocclusions. Questions have been alluded to with reference to enlarging the upper jaw and straightening of the teeth. Again, any oral or plastic surgical procedure on the upper jaw or palate is impractical because of the malrelationship of the entire midface maldevelopment and supporting cranial structure. Orthodontic considerations must, however, be highly individualized according to both patient and professional.

The malformations seen in the teeth do not cause any appreciable problems. Dental health care and hygiene must be given high priority to ensure retention of the teeth. Even though the instances of dental caries are few, regulation of diet and nutrition is of considerable value in keeping the caries activity down and yet increasing the resistance of the gums to periodontal disease, which is seen quite frequently in these patients. Bruxism can cause loosening and early exfoliation of the teeth. This should be controlled through a behavior modification and early stimulation program to eliminate this destructive habit.

DISCUSSION

A review of the basic facial and oral manifestations of persons with Down's Syndrome has been presented. It can be seen that many of these manifestations, or characteristics, do overlap and contribute to influencing factors on other characteristics. To understand the facial features and the facial posture of these individuals one must consider not the separate areas or compartments, but rather the complex structure which is comprised of many smaller, basic units. These basic structures form the foundation on which we can build a sophisticated human model system, such as the face, with its many functions and movements. Understanding the deficiencies of these basic structures is paramount to understanding the complexities and complicated interactions that comprise the human face in persons who have an inherent insult to the genesis and maturation of these basic structures. These structures may be influenced by the chromosomal abnormality which contributes to growth and development of the cells in these structural units. The face and oral structure of the individual with Down's Syndrome is malformed because of a deficiency in some of the basic structural units that make up the craniofacial complex. It is difficult to build that which is complex when the basic foundation is deficient in potential development.

REFERENCES

1. SPITZER, R.: Observations on congenital dentofacial disorders in mongolism and microcephaly. *Oral Surgery* 24:325, 1967.
2. GORLIN, R. J.: Chromosomal abnormalities and oral anomalies. *J. Dent. Res.* 42:1297, 1963.
3. GOODMAN, R. M., and GORLIN, R. J.: *The Face in Genetic Disorders.* St. Louis: C. V. Mosby, 1970.
4. SEWARD, F. S., ROCHE, A. F. and SUNDERLAND, S.: The lateral cranial silhouette in mongolism. *Amer. J. Roentgenol.* 85:653, 1961.
5. FROSTAD, N. A., CLEALL, J. F. and MELOSKY, C. C.: Craniofacial complex in the trisomy 21 syndrome (Down's Syndrome). *Arch. Oral. Biol.* 16:707, 1971.
6. OSTER, J.: *Mongolism.* Copenhagen: Danish Science Press, Ltd., 1953.
7. GOSMAN, S. D.: Facial development in mongolism. *Amer. J. Orthodont.* 37:332, 1951.
8. COHEN, M. M., and WINER, R. A.: Dental and facial characteristics in Down's Syndrome (mongolism). *J. Dent. Res.* 44:197, 1965.
9. BENDA, C. E.: *The Child with Mongolism (Congenital Acromicria).* New York: Grune and Stratton, 1960.
10. ROCHE, A. F., ROCHE, P. J., and LEWIS, A. B.: The cranial base in trisomy 21. *J. Ment. Defic. Res.* 16:7, 1972.
11. CUMMINS, H., TALLEY, C., and PLATOU, R. V.: Palmar dermatoglyphics in mongolism. *Pediatrics* 5:241, 1950.

12. LEVINSON, A., FRIEDMAN, A., and STAMPS, F.: Variability of mongolism. *Pediatrics* 16:43, 1955.
13. SHAPIRO, B. L., GORLIN, R. J., REDMAN, R. S., and BRUHL, H. H.: The palate and Down's Syndrome. *New Engl. J. Med.* 276:1460, 1967.
14. ARDRAN, G. M., HARKER, P., and KEMP, F. H.: Tongue size in Down's Syndrome. *J. Ment. Defic. Res.* 16:160, 1972.
15. JOHNSON, N. P., and YOUNG, M. A.: Periodontal disease in mongols. *J. Perio.* 34:41, 1963.
16. COHEN, M. M., WINER, R. A., SCHWARTZ, S., and SHKLAR, G.: Oral aspects of mongolism. *Oral Surgery* 14:92, 1961.
17. BROWN, R. H., and CUNNINGHAM, W. M. Some dental manifestations of mongolism. *Oral Surgery* 14:664, 1961.
18. GULLIKSON, J. S.: Oral findings in children with Down's Syndrome. *J. Dent. Child.* 60:293, 1973.
19. COHEN, M. M., Sr., and COHEN, M. M., Jr.: Oral manifestations of trisomy Gl (Down's Syndrome). *Birth Defects, Original Article Series,* Vol. VII: 7,241, 1971.
20. WINER, R. A., COHEN, M. M., FELLER, R. P., and CHAUNCY, H. H.: Comparison of human saliva, secretory rate, and electrolyte concentration in mentally subnormal persons. *J. Dent. Res.* 44:632, 1965.
21. WINER, R. A., and FELLER, R. P.: Comparison of parotid and submandibular saliva and serum in Down's Syndrome. *J. Dent. Res.* 51:449, 1972.
22. ROCHE. A. F., and BARKLA, D. H.: The eruption of deciduous teeth in mongols. *J. Ment. Defic. Res.* 8:54, 1964.
23. BARKLA, D. H.: Ages of eruption of permanent teeth in mongols. *J. Ment. Defic. Res.* 10:190, 1966.
24. MCMILLIAN, R. S., and KASHGARIAN, M.: Relation of human abnormalities of structure and function to abnormalities of the dentition, II mongolism. *J. Amer. Dent. Ass.* 63:368, 1961.
25. INGALLS, T. H., and BUTLER, R. L.: Mongolism: Implications of dental anomalies. *New Engl. J. Med.* 248:511, 1953.
26. COHEN, M. M., BLITZER, F. J., ARVYSTAS, M. G., and BONNEAU, R. H.: Abnormalities of the permanent dentition in Down's Syndrome (mongolism). *J. Dent. Res.* 49:1386, 1970.
27. MESKIN, L. H., and GORLIN, R. J.: Agenesis and peg-shaped permanent maxillary lateral incisors. *J. Dent. Res.* 42:1476, 1963.
28. GECIAUSKAS, M. A., and COHEN, M. M.: Mesiodistal crown diameter of permanent teeth in Down's Syndrome (mongolism). *Amer. J. Ment. Defic.* 74:503, 1970.
29. COHEN, M. M., ARVYSTAS, M. G., and BAUM, B. J.: Occlusal disharmonies in trisomy G (Down's Syndrome, mongolism). *Amer. J. Orthodont.* 58:367, 1970.

5

Prenatal Detection of Down's Syndrome: Technical and Ethical Considerations

MICHAEL M. KABACK, M.D. *and*

JAAKKO LEISTI, M.D.

The interaction between health professionals and lay organizations is essential since we are all working toward the same goal—improvement in the quality of life for children and families where serious birth defects have occurred. In this instance we are emphasizing a specific and serious disorder, Down's Syndrome.

It is important to initiate our remarks in an historical perspective since there has been a virtual revolution in biomedical sciences in the last two decades. Recent technological advances have raised enormous and important new issues with implications for our generation and generations to come. For this reason it is imperative that people throughout our society, representing various disciplines and perspectives, consider these new technologies and how they may be implemented to best benefit individuals and families within our society, as well as the society at large.

The technology developed through basic research in the last 20 years now enables us to consider the possibility of prevention and control of human genetic disease. New information developed from

Supported in part by NIH Graduate Research Training Grant (HD 00417), NICHD contract—(National Registry for Amniocentesis), and Grant Awards from the National Foundation—March of Dimes, and the Southeast Association for Retarded Children.

laboratories all over the world has led to new capabilities and new clinical tools which, if appropriately and wisely utilized, can benefit many people in our society.

Some of these new capabilities have raised the possibility of effective control for certain human genetic disorders (1). Control could be envisioned by one of three mechanisms: a disease might be controlled if it could be cured, if it could be effectively treated, or if it could be prevented.

In considering these approaches, it is clear that our scientific capabilities are still quite limited and that our ignorance still far exceeds our knowledge. Accordingly, at this time and in light of current knowledge, it is unrealistic and infeasible to contemplate a complete cure for a disorder like Down's Syndrome. Many people read the important medical literature of our time in places like the *Ladies Home Journal* and *Reader's Digest,* and are aware of the almost magical words "genetic engineering in the *cure* of human genetic disease." As medical geneticists, we have reservations about the immediacy of any of these applications and feel that it is inappropriate to spend a great deal of time considering these futuristic concepts now.

On the other hand, enormous breakthroughs have been made, and continue to be made, in the area of *effective treatment* of genetic disease. Certainly there are many, many human genetic abnormalities which can now be effectively treated so that the genetically affected individual can live an essentially normal life. Phenylketonuria, galactosemia, and other diseases of this type can now be effectively treated if they are diagnosed early and treatment is initiated early in life. Unfortunately, with Down's Syndrome, we are not that far as yet, but important efforts continue in this direction.

It is the *prevention* of serious genetic disease which we would like to consider in depth here, mainly because this is an approach which offers many families an important alternative today which did not exist just a few years ago.

It is important to emphasize that where new technology is to be utilized, it must be done so on an individualized basis—and that sweeping general applications must be avoided. Technology itself does not pose questions of an ethical or moral nature. It is the application of technology that raises such questions. We would like to consider the technology of prenatal diagnosis, particularly as it relates to the prevention of Down's Syndrome, and to consider some of the positive as well as negative implications.

Certainly one of the areas where the greatest strides have been made in the field of human genetics relates to the ability to cultivate human cells and to study them in the laboratory. Using a small amount of peripheral blood or a tiny skin biopsy, we can now grow large numbers of human cells in the laboratory and, from them, characterize the chromosomal make-up and many of the genetic characteristics of the individual from whom the cells originate. This provides a remarkable opportunity to study human biology in the laboratory. A tiny skin biopsy the size of a match head, if grown to its maximum potential, would yield approximately 300-400 pounds of cells, every one of which would continue to reflect the genetic constitution of the individual from whom the skin fragment was originally taken. This technique provides an opportunity to study human genetic mechanisms not in the person himself, but rather in a culture of his or her cells grown in the laboratory.

The cultivation of these cells involves the ubiquitous biological process of mitosis—the process by which one cell divides into two (Figure 1). There is a great deal that we do not yet know about this very primary process of living matter, although it is, perhaps, in this process that the answer to the problem of Down's Syndrome lies. But an enormous amount of research is needed if that answer is to be found. With this kind of laboratory capability, however, we can, in fact, begin to look at such processes in detail.

INTRAUTERINE DIAGNOSIS

Amniocentesis is the obstetrical procedure used in the intrauterine detection of genetic disease. Simply stated, the fetus, *in utero,* grows within a sac of amniotic fluid. It has been known for many years that all fetuses, as they grow in this sac of fluid, shed cells from their skin, from the membranes around them, from their mouth,

FIGURE 1

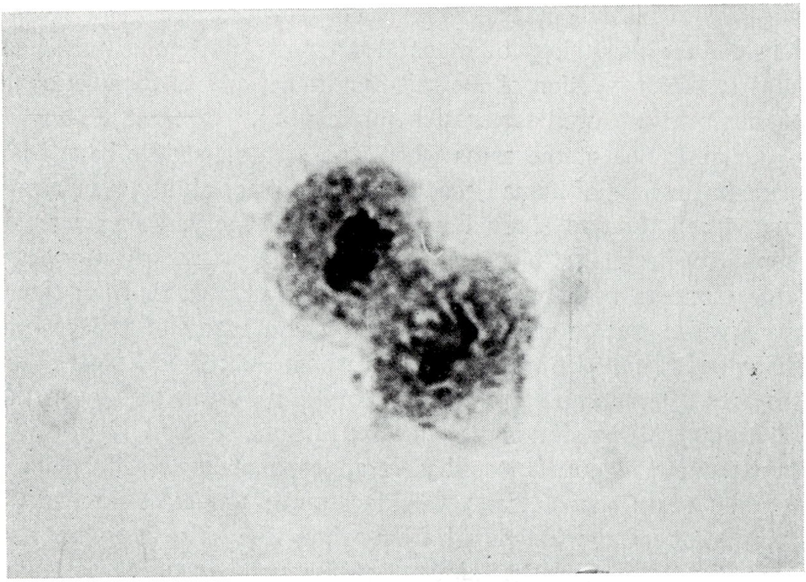

A fibroblastic cell in mitosis. The dark bodies within the cells are the chromosomes separating during cellular division. When this process is complete, two independent cells will result.

from their genito-urinary tract, and possibly from multiple other sites in the fetal organism. It has also been known for some time that one can obtain small samples of amniotic fluid by placing a needle into the sac (amniocentesis); but it was not until the mid 1960's that the implications of this technique for the detection and prevention of certain human genetic diseases really became apparent (2). It is now clear that with a high degree of safety and accuracy, amniocentesis can be performed during the third or fourth month of pregnancy to obtain a small sample of amniotic fluid. Most recently, the use of ultrasonic scanning of the women's abdomen (using a sound detector system) prior to the amniocentesis has aided the obstetrician in avoiding the placenta and fetus to further minimize the risks of the procedure.

Amniocentesis involves the use of a needle about the same width

FIGURE 2

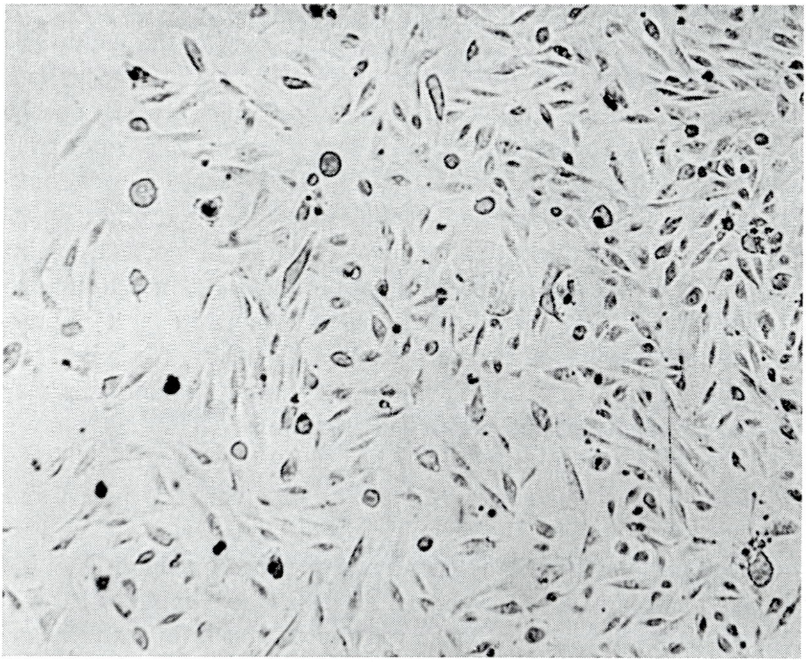

Amniotic fluid cells (of fetal origin) in culture 7 days after amniocentesis. A variety of cell types are evident. The round cells represent dividing cells, i.e. undergoing mitosis.

as that which is used for a penicillin injection. The needle is introduced through the skin of the middle abdomen, through the uterine muscle, and into the uterine sac. Then a small sample of straw-colored fluid (the amniotic fluid) is removed. The fetal cells are then collected from the fluid (by centrifugation) and placed in special nutrient medium under carefully defined conditions in the cell culture laboratory. Figure 2 shows what these cells look like after being cultured for about 7-10 days. These are cells growing under the microscope, where we can observe them and evaluate a number of specific genetic parameters of these growing cells *in vitro*. From these analyses, as from the growing skin or blood cells of postnatal individuals, we can ascertain a number of facts about the genetic constitution of the fetus.

This new and exciting technology, coupled with the continuing evolution in social and ethical attitudes of our society, opens new doors for medical science—but these are doors which must be opened with great care and concern. With current techniques approximately 30 to 40 serious genetic disorders, as well as most chromosomal abnormalities, can be detected in the fetus (3). Unfortunately, we cannot, as yet, effectively treat or correct such problems. The family, however, can gain important information about the health of their fetus and can, if they so choose, electively terminate (abort) a pregnancy where an affected fetus is identified. Certainly this is far from a perfect solution to the problem, but for many families this may provide an important and positive alternative.

For centuries, the fetus has been "off limits" to the medical scientist. But now, with advancing technology, this taboo has been lifted. Fetology is now within the new domain of medical science, and we may soon not only be able to detect and prevent genetic disease, but we may be able to treat or correct fetal disorders *in utero* as well. With further research it is hoped we may be able to initiate therapy for certain disorders early in fetal life or even to perform corrective surgical procedures on the fetus as can be done on certain other mammalian species now. Obviously, in this context, the ability to accurately diagnose specific fetal disease is the absolute prerequisite to such future treatment or correction programs. Accordingly, continued support for research directed at improved fetal diagnosis provides the foundation upon which future treatment and correction programs will be built.

CHROMOSOME DISORDERS

Individuals *born* with abnormal chromosome constitutions represent the very tip of the iceberg of chromosome abnormalities. A number of studies have been done in recent years to evaluate the causes of spontaneous abortions in early pregnancy, and it has become quite apparent that chromosomal anomalies—being present in

TABLE 1

Percentage of Chromosome Anomalies in 220 Spontaneous Abortions

Menstrual Age	% Of Fetuses With Chromosome Anomaly
< 13 weeks	40%
13-17 weeks	25%
> 17 weeks	3.5%

derived from data of Carr, 1970(4).

from 35% to 50% of the aborted fetuses—form the most important causative group (4, 5). Table 1 is a summary of data from a large series of spontaneous abortions and the results of chromosome analyses performed. All these fetuses resulted from spontaneous termination of pregnancy; no amniocentesis procedure was performed.

If one looks at the chromosome constitution of the aborted fetus as a function of gestational age, it is apparent that the sooner the pregnancy ends in abortion, the higher is the frequency of chromosome anomalies. In fetuses spontaneously aborted before 13 weeks of pregnancy the frequency is as high as 40%, while in abortions occurring after 17 weeks of pregnancy the incidence has dropped to 3.5%. The chromosome anomalies include duplicate sets of chromosomes, absence of chromosomes and chromosomal trisomies including trisomy 21, which causes Down's Syndrome. Interestingly, it has been estimated that 63% of fetuses with trisomy G abort early in pregnancy (6). It is important to appreciate that nature, to a large degree, selects against chromosome abnormalities (including Down's Syndrome) by the mechanism of spontaneous abortion (see Table 2). With this background intrauterine diagnosis and the elective abortion of a chromosomally abnormal fetus may take on a different light.

What do we know about the chromosome abnormalities that do survive pregnancy? Table 3 shows the frequency of a series of chromosome aberrations at birth.

It is clear from a number of surveys in various parts of the world that about 1 in 600 children born has Down's Syndrome or mon-

TABLE 2

Estimates of Autosomal Trisomies Among Conceptions which Implant and an Estimate of Prenatal Loss*

	In All Conceptions†	In Live Newborns	Prenatal Loss
Trisomy D	0.35%	0.02%	91%
Trisomy E	0.56%	0.02%	96%
Trisomy G	0.48%	0.15%**	63%

† Based on assumption that 15% of all implanted conceptions abort
* derived from data of Hamerton, 1971(6).
** Trisomy 21

TABLE 3

Observed Frequencies of Major Chromosome Anomalies in Newborn Infants

Chromosome Anomaly	Frequency
Trisomy 13	1: 4000 - 8000 births
Trisomy 18	1: 4000 - 8000 births
Trisomy 21	1: 670 births
XXY	1: 830 male births
XYY	1: 660 male births
XXX	1: 1500 female births
XO	1: 2500 female births

derived from collected data of Hamerton, 1971(6).

golism. This is certainly one of the most frequent, if not *the* most frequent, chromosomal abnormality which survives pregnancy.

The impact of Down's Syndrome on families varies a great deal. Mrs. Rockefeller's comments in this volume are enormously relevant to this point. As pediatrician-geneticists we have worked closely with families in which a child with Down's Syndrome has occurred and where great joy and love have been shared in both directions. Certainly this could in no way be considered a tragedy. But, quite honestly, in many families the birth of a child with Down's Syndrome has been a tragic event.

Tragic in what sense?—tragic for the Down's Syndrome child in that particular family, for the healthy siblings of the child, for the parents, for other family members, and, to a certain degree, tragic for the community at large as well. It is that kind of "mass tragedy" that can now be prevented with some of the new technology at hand. Down's Syndrome in a child need not be a tragedy, but where it would likely be, the prevention of that tragedy for so many individuals (including perhaps the Down's Syndrome child himself) is worthy of consideration.

A CASE IN POINT

These concepts can be best exemplified perhaps by a family we dealt with several years ago at our center. The first child born to this young couple (father 27, mother 25) was identified in the delivery room to have many of the stigmata of Down's Syndrome. The child was also one of the 35% of mongoloid individuals with congenital heart disease, in this case, a serious defect with an opening between all four chambers of the heart. Chromosomal analysis of this child revealed that the child had the translocation type of Down's Syndrome (Figure 3).

Here, the number of chromosomes in each of the child's cells was 46 (as in normal individuals), but an unusual chromosome was identified in which an extra 21 chromosome was attached to a number 13 chromosome. So this child actually had an extra 21 chromosome and was clinically, therefore, the same as the usual trisomy 21 Down's Syndrome (in which 47 chromosomes are found in each cell).

Chromosomal analysis of the parents showed the father to have a normal complement of 46 chromosomes but the mother's cells contained only 45 chromosomes. However it was shown that the mother also had the "translocated" (double) chromosome. Therefore she had the proper amount of chromosomal and genetic material but two of her chromosomes were attached together. This was of no significance as far as her own health is concerned, but was vitally important with regard to her reproductive potential.

Based on these findings we could predict for this young family that they would have approximately a 10 to 20% risk that each pregnancy which reached term would result in another Down's Syndrome

FIGURE 3

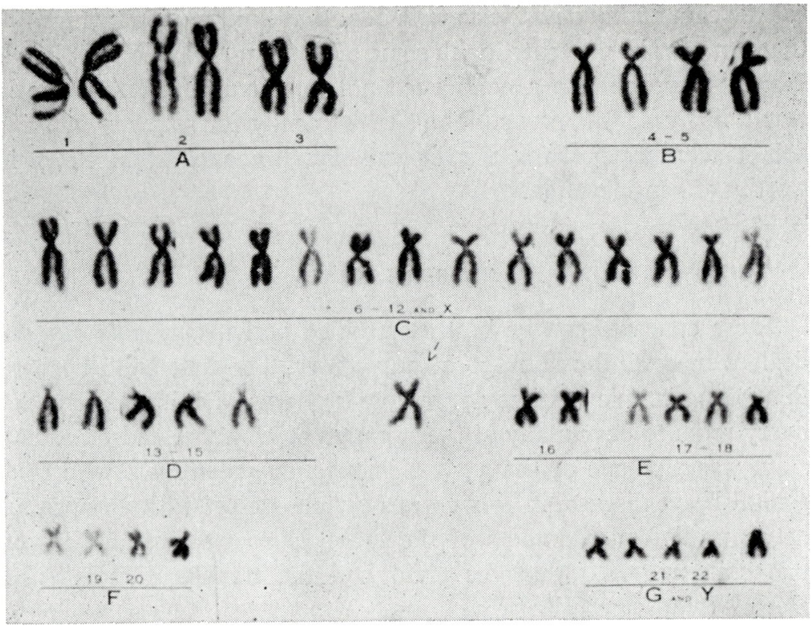

Karyotype of the patient with Down's Syndrome. Notice that the extra chromosome #21 has attached to a D-group chromosome (indicated by arrow), and that the total number of chromosomes is 46.

child. They were also informed that their risk for spontaneous abortion with each conception might be as high as 25% as well.

Their Down's Syndrome child was quite ill throughout his first two years of life. He suffered many respiratory infections, went into heart failure several times, and required hospitalization on five separate occasions. He died at 2½ years of age. For this unsuspecting young couple this was not only a devastating emotional experience, but an enormous financial burden as well. This family, after a great deal of thought and consideration, decided that they would not risk having more children because they were fearful of having another child with Down's Syndrome. The increasing strain on their relationship became apparent in subsequent counseling sessions with each of them individually and together as a couple.

FIGURE 4

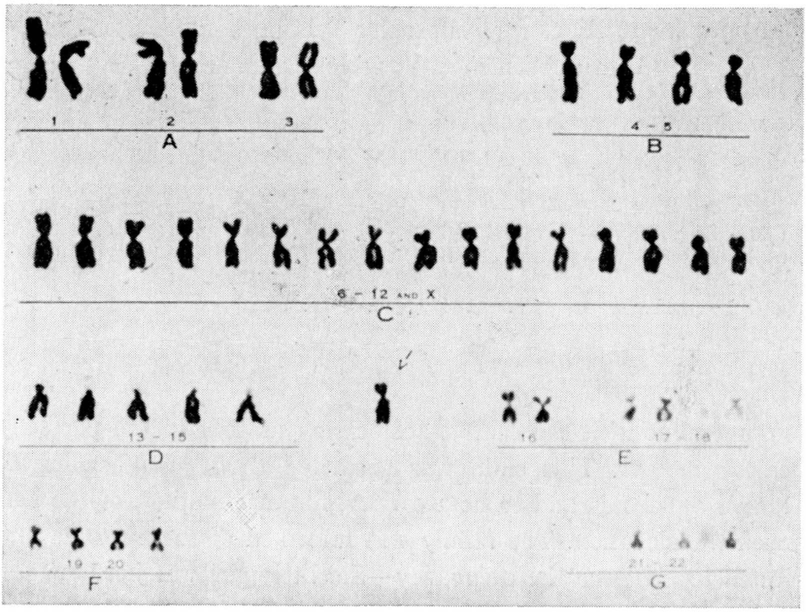

Karyotype derived from amniotic fluid cells obtained from a subsequent pregnancy in the mother of patient (Fig. 3). This illustrates the balanced translocation state in which a #21 chromosome is attached to a D-group chromosome. There are 45 apparent chromosomes, but one represents a double chromosome (#21 - #13 - indicated by arrow). This child remains entirely normal at age 3½. An identical karyotype was found in the healthy mother.

It was just about this time that the clinical applicability of prenatal genetic diagnosis began to emerge. Within a year our facilities were established and we were confident of our ability to perform amniocentesis, to grow fetal cells, and to accurately assess the chromosomal complement of the growing fetal cells. The family was informed of this new capability and the issues of prenatal diagnostic technology were discussed in detail with them. They decided to try another pregnancy.

The next figure (Figure 4) shows the analysis of fetal chromosomes from amniotic cells completed after the amniocentesis in their next pregnancy. A female fetus was identified who had only 45 chro-

TABLE 4

Approximate Risks for Autosomal Trisomies in Live Infants Born to Women of Varying Maternal Age

Maternal Age	Trisomy 13	Trisomy 18	Trisomy 21
< 19 yrs.	1:13,500	1: 5,750	
20 - 24 yrs.	1: 7,830	1: 5,551	1: 3,600
25 - 29 yrs.	1: 9,100	1: 3,120	1: 3,000
30 - 34 yrs.	1: 7,150	1: 4,380	1: 580
35 - 39 yrs.	1: 2,080	1: 2,601	1: 280
40 - 44 yrs.	1: 674	1: 553	1: 70
45 > yrs.	1: 134	1: 229	1: 38

mosomes but with the same translocation as that of the perfectly healthy mother. This child was predicted to be unaffected with Down's Syndrome and to be a carrier, like her mother, of the balanced translocation. The family was informed of these results and elected to continue the pregnancy—the little girl was born several months later. She is now about 3½ or 4 years of age and is a beautiful and bright little girl. This family has since had another pregnancy which also resulted in an unaffected child who is now 2 years old and healthy.

This is what amniocentesis and prenatal diagnosis are really about. They are not, in our consideration, about the abortion of Down's Syndrome fetuses. They are about the health and life of children who might never have been born, at least to some families, if this capability did not exist. Certainly this consideration has to be highly individualized; not all families would accept amniocentesis and possible abortion of pregnancy on personal or religious grounds. Such an attitude is only to be respected. But, for other families who would be fearful of even considering reproduction, and who could accept elective abortion where the fetus would have a serious and untreatable genetic disorder, this alternative provides a meaningful and positive approach for them to have children and to achieve their hopes for having offspring.

GENETIC CONSIDERATIONS AND RECENT EXPERIENCE

There are other aspects of Down's Syndrome which are well recognized. Table 4 shows the incidence of trisomies 13, 18 and 21, as a function of the age of the mother at the time of pregnancy. The incidence of trisomy 21 (Down's Syndrome) dramatically increases in the offspring of women who become pregnant after the age of 35 years (although the absolute risks are still quite small). The same phenomenon occurs with the other major trisomies as well. In fact, for all of the nondisjunction-type of chromosome abnormalities (of which Down's Syndrome is a prime example) increased maternal age increases the risk of such chromosome aberrations occurring in the offspring.

This phenomenon is also observed with the sex chromosome abnormalities as well. For Klinefelter syndrome (XXY) and Triplo-X (XXX) a similar increase in incidence is seen with advanced maternal age. For Turner's syndrome (XO), an age related increase in incidence is not seen. Increased paternal age has been shown not to increase the risk for Down's Syndrome, but does for several other genetic disorders.

Since 1967, over 2000 pregnancies have been monitored during the second trimester by amniocentesis in North America (7). Nearly 80% of these have been done because of a risk for chromosomal disorders in the fetus. The major categories include women of advanced maternal age (greater than 35-40), women who have had a trisomy 21 child previously, and women in families where one or the other parent was a carrier of a balanced translocation.

Of the first 600 women over 35 who had their pregnancies tested, 21 of the fetuses were found to have chromosomal abnormalities. This represents a frequency of 3.5%. In essentially every instance, the couple, when informed of the abnormal chromosome status of their fetus, elected to abort the pregnancy. In the other 96.5% of these families, they could be assured that their fetus would not have a chromosomal derangement and their fears and anxieties were completely allayed.

Some very important data have come forth from the first 450 amniocenteses done in women under 35 who had had a previous G-trisomy child. There has been a debate over the years among geneticists as to what the recurrence risk is for such women. It had been estimated that the risk would be no greater than that observed in women of the same age without a previous child with mongolism. The fact that they already had one child with Down's Syndrome would not increase the risk for subsequent children with Down's Syndrome. Others found families in which multiple cases of 21 trisomy occurred. A new and empirical risk figure was arrived at which suggested that a woman's chances of giving birth to another child with Down's Syndrome were perhaps twice that of a woman of her age who had not previously delivered a mongoloid baby. That is, if a 30-year-old woman with no previous history has a one in 1,000 chance of having a mongoloid child, a woman who has already had a Down's Syndrome child and then becomes pregnant at 30 might have a risk of one in 500 rather than one in 1,000. This question has been considered in a number of retrospective studies. But now through amniocentesis we can look at the fetus before it reaches term, and thereby begin to collect new and prospective information. In the monitored pregnancies of women where a mongoloid child had been born previously, amniocentesis indicated the recurrence of trisomy 21 in the fetus at the third or fourth month of pregnancy in 5 of 500 pregnancies. A one percent risk figure, or one in 100, is probably a more accurate figure than the probabilities that had been previously quoted.

With parental balanced translocation, as we would have predicted, nearly 20% of the pregnancies were found to have the unbalanced chromosomal abnormality associated with Down's Syndrome. In almost every such instance, the families elected to terminate the pregnancy. Where the *balanced* translocation carrier fetus was identified, as far as we know, no family elected to terminate the pregnancy; nor could we understand a reason for doing so since the child would be perfectly healthy and normal, but simply carry the chromosomal translocation.

In general, then, the great majority of pregnancies where amniocentesis has been applied have resulted in the term delivery of normal, healthy children. In the very small number of instances where a chromosomal abnormality was identified, the families were informed thoroughly and made their own decisions as to how to proceed. Most, if not all, elected to abort the pregnancy. Importantly, however, many of the healthy children born might never have been conceived or reached delivery without intrauterine diagnosis to help their families. More children have been born as the result of prenatal diagnosis than would have been born without it, and the children are a great deal healthier.

RISKS OF AMNIOCENTESIS

What is the risk of amniocentesis? This is a critical question since we may be dealing with a family in which the risk may be only one percent for having a child with an abnormality. Wouldn't the risk of the procedure affect the decision whether or not to have the procedure done? We do not yet have an absolute figure for the overall risks of amniocentesis, but one could certainly list a whole series of *potential complications* associated with amniocentesis. There might be problems for the fetus or the mother in the immediate time period surrounding the procedure (hemorrhage, infection, spontaneous labor and loss of pregnancy, etc.). A second group of potential problems relates to the prenatal and perinatal periods: could amniocentesis affect the fetus in its development during the rest of the pregnancy; would the prematurity rate be increased; or would problems in the newborn period be increased? A third group of potential complications relates to long-term problems, e.g., whether or not removing a small sample of fluid from the pregnant uterus might incur any damage to the fetus throughout its subsequent life.

We have been carefully looking for such complications but this procedure is very new and we really have a relatively small sample of pregnancies in which to evaluate these kinds of questions. To appropriately evaluate these issues we must have data about the incidence of spontaneous abortion or other problems in this trimester and about the spontaneous incidence of growth retardation in late trimester pregnancies, for example. These questions must be resolved if we are to really evaluate whether or not amniocentesis is causing such problems.

At this point it is appropriate to indicate that the reported frequency of any complications with amniocentesis is around two percent, but the great majority of these were minor complications which neither caused the pregnancy to end nor caused any serious or obvious problem. The women may have leaked amniotic fluid for a few days or there may have been a small amount of vaginal spotting, but the pregnancies went on to term resulting in normal and healthy newborns. There have been about six or seven spontaneous labor and abortions within 3 weeks following amniocentesis (from a group of about 1500 studied). That is a very small proportion. A certain number of those abortions might have occurred even if amniocentesis had not been done. It is really too early to give an absolute answer to the overall risks but we can say with certainty that the serious complication rate of amniocentesis, particularly the immediate or short-term complication frequency, is not greater than one percent, that is 1 in 100 pregnancies.

The National Institute of Child Health and Human Development is currently sponsoring a program in this country in which nine centers are involved in a collaborative, prospective study to critically define the risks of amniocentesis. The results of this study will be completed in about one year. In this study, each time a woman, in concurrence with her husband, elects to have a pregnancy monitored by amniocentesis, she is matched with one, or preferably two, women who are also pregnant and of comparable age, race, previous pregnancies, etc. The two women who are matched as controls are not having amniocentesis done in their pregnancy. The amniocentesis case and the non-amniocentesis cases are then evaluated in exactly the same fashion for the remainder of their pregnancies. The comparison goes through the newborn period and includes careful monitoring of development and health status of the babies from birth through their first year of life. It is only in this way that we will be able to develop more accurate data on the overall risks of amniocentesis.

In the many centers throughout this country (and others) where prenatal diagnosis is conducted, the accuracy of the method has proven to be incredibly high. Like any medical procedure or test, answers are not *always* correct or obtainable but with intrauterine genetic testing, the accuracy is greater than 99%. This is a great credit to the laboratories involved and reflects the great concern and care with which these delicate tests are conducted.

ETHICAL CONSIDERATIONS

Much has been said and written about the implications of this new procedure. A number of sensitive ethical, moral, and legal questions have been raised. We have alluded to certain aspects of these issues. While the selective abortion of fetuses with serious genetic disease can be debated ethically, prenatal diagnosis has been of enormous positive human value for the many families who have chosen to use this new alternative. We have considered this a "positive alternative" in genetic counseling because it can enable many couples, who find this approach acceptable, to reproduce without fear; as we have indicated, the fear of recurrence of Down's Syndrome or other serious genetic disease has prohibited certain families from trying to have further children. Unfortunately, in many instances this has led to family disruption, separation, divorce, and so forth. Because this "positive alternative" is now available to such families, they can still have children without fear of such conditions in subsequent children.

Whose right is it to make such decisions? In our opinion, it should be the individual family's right to make that decision. Not every family in which the woman is over 35 and becomes pregnant should have an amniocentesis, but we strongly believe that every such family should know about amniocentesis, should understand what the risks are, and should be able to make their own decision as to whether or not to have an amniocentesis. Further, the decision as to what they would do if an abnormality were detected is also best made by the individual family along with their physician. For many families, additional counsel might be sought from their religious leader, from other family members, etc. Ultimately, the decision must be made by the parents, at least in terms of current social attitudes.

What are the rights of the fetus? Many have argued that no one represents the fetus in such decisions. This is, needless to say, a very delicate question. But on the other hand, if one wants to raise ethical questions, perhaps the fetus would make choices if it could, and who is to know what choice it would make if it knew the limitation of its life potential and the impact of its life on that particular family.

Some have argued that intrauterine diagnosis and selective abortion are the same as euthanasia. But there are enormous differences between abortion and euthanasia—not so much in biological or scientific terms, but certainly in terms of the human psyche and attitudes toward children and the definition of life. Terminating a pregnancy before a woman has identified, in any real sense, with the fetus is very different from taking the life of an infant whom a woman has carried to term, made detailed plans for, delivered, and felt a true closeness to.

The basic question that much of this technology raises is: "As our technology to detect imperfection improves, will society's tolerance for imperfection become less and less?" This is a question which all of us have to begin thinking about because our technology is improving and moving ahead rapidly. Who defines the level of imperfection that is or is not acceptable? These are very basic ethical questions which society must think about.

We are developing a capability now which will allow us to look directly at the fetus with a "fetoscope" early in pregnancy and to obtain blood or tissue samples from the fetus *in utero*. Ultimately, this may lead to methods for the treatment of disease very early in fetal existence. We must consider these new technologies not only in terms of prevention through abortion but also in terms of a real approach to treatment or even cure of some of these conditions in the future.

What other current dilemmas do we face? If people want to make choices as to whether to have male or female children, should technology be applied to such a goal? We think not. Our position is that we are willing to use this technology to aid a family, a *selected* family, in the prevention of a tragic genetic disease. It is not, in our judgment, a tragic genetic disease if a child is of the "wrong" sex, according to the parents' desires. The decision to abort a pregnancy on the basis of the fetus being a boy or a girl is, in our opinion, a misuse of technology.

What are the future implications to society of these new technologies? If carefully utilized, they would have a very minimal effect on future generations in terms of decreasing the frequency of deleterious genes or on chromosome carrier states of the type that we have discussed. The ultimate question is: "Who has the right to make these decisions?" The decision is not one that should be imposed on anyone. We strongly resist the idea that legislatures, whether they be federal, local or state, should make amniocentesis and prevention of genetic disease mandatory.

On the other hand, the government can play an important role in providing support for education, not only to married couples, but perhaps to children as well, concerning the basic facts of human genetics and human genetic disorders. In this way our population will learn that human beings have genes and chromosomes, and there are means, when these chromosomes and genes are arranged abnormally, to detect and thereby control the problem prenatally.

We shall end our discussion with this last point, because it is the ultimate decision which is really the major question of all this technology. It we use our technology in a way that will benefit the individual, the family, and the society as a whole, then it will be well utilized. If we use it otherwise, it may cause greater problems than it solves. It is very much our feeling that the growing technology can be used now, in individualized instances, to help families minimize the tragedy of untreatable genetic disease and maximize the joy of healthy children. It is our hope, however, that the dilemmas of today's technology will be resolved through continued research and discovery and through an expanded enlightenment throughout our society.

REFERENCES

1. KABACK, M. M.: Perspectives in the Control of Human Genetic Disease. *Genetics and the Perinatal Patient.* Mead Johnson Symposium on Perinatal and Developmental Medicine, No. I. Vail, Colorado, 1972.
2. NADLER, H. L.: Prenatal Detection of Genetic Defects. *J. Pediat.* 74: 132-143, 1968.
3. BURTON, B. K., GERBIE, A. B. and NADLER, H. L.: Present status of Intrauterine Diagnosis of Genetic Defects. *Am. J. Obstet. Gynecol.* 118: 718-746, 1974.

4. CARR, D. H.: Chromosome Abnormalities and Spontaneous Abortions. *Human Population Cytogenetics*, Eds. P. A. Jacobs, W. H. Price & P. Law, pp. 103-118, Edinburgh, Scotland: Edinburgh University Press, 1970.
5. BOUE, J-G, and BOUE, A: Les Aberrations Chromosomiques Dans Les Avortements Spontanés Humains. *Presse Med.* 78: 635-641, 1970.
6. HAMERTON, J. L.: Human cytogenetics. *Clinical Cytogenetics* Vol. II, New York: Academic Press, 1971.
7. MILUNSKY, A.: *The Prenatal Diagnosis of Hereditary Disorders.* Springfield, Illinois. Charles C. Thomas, 1973.

6

Family Planning as a Method of Prevention

ZENA A. STEIN, M.A., M.B., B.CH.

New approaches, in particular, prenatal diagnosis, relating to the preventability of Down's Syndrome, raise fundamental issues for public health and social action. Let's start by describing some population characteristics of Down's Syndrome which need to be taken into consideration in relation to family planning and prevention.

First, with regard to incidence, i.e. the new cases that arise over a period of time, the population factor that has most to do with the rate of occurrence of Down's Syndrome at birth is maternal age. Older women bear more children with Down's Syndrome than younger women. The relative fertility of older to younger women in the population, therefore, directly determines incidence.

As an example, we applied the known risk factors for Down's Syndrome, for each maternal age, to estimate the number of children with Down's Syndrome that would have been born each year from 1953 to 1970 in New York City. The actual number of Down's Syndrome infants born, according to our calculations, fell from about 200 in 1950 to about 150 in 1970. This represents a decrease of 25 percent. However, since the total number of births also fell over that period the incidence rate, which is the proportion of Down's Syndrome among all babies, fell only 11 percent, from 1.25 per 1000 to about 1.1 per 1000 (1, 2).

Most of the reduction in incidence resulted from the fact that the number of older women living in New York City had declined. On the other hand, the reduction in incidence contributed by a reduction in the fertility of older women through family planning, etc., changed little over the same period. This means that the incidence rate is probably not changing very much.

By contrast, the prevalence of Down's Syndrome has risen steeply over the last few decades, and it is probably still rising. This prevalence indicates the proportion of individuals who have the condition, compared to the whole population at a given time. It is the real rate for which the community must plan. Prevalence defines the minimal need for educational, health, welfare, and family resources.

Not only has the prevalence of Down's Syndrome been rising, but it has been doing so at a time when other conditions known to cause severe mental retardation have been declining. Tuberculosis, syphilis, cretinisn and phenylketonuria are well established examples of such causes. The changing importance of Down's Syndrome among the causes of severe mental retardation is a dramatic historic fact. The British authority, Tredgold, wrote in 1940 (3): "The number of Mongols is not large. They probably do not form more than 4 or 5 percent of all aments." Most current surveys show a far higher percent of Down's Syndrome among the severely retarded, sometimes as high as 25 percent.

There is no mystery to this rising prevalence. There has been an absolute rise over a period of time, due to an increased expectation of life in the persons affected. Between 1940 and 1960, the life expectancy at birth of persons with Down's Syndrome is estimated to have risen from about 12 to about 16 years. Approximately one-half of the infants with Down's Syndrome now survive the respiratory diseases to which they were particularly likely to succumb in the past. Except for certain malformations and leukemia (from which about one percent of the persons with Down's Syndrome die), the once fatal hazards common among these children are becoming amenable to treatment. Surgery corrects congenital abnormalities, vaccines protect against a growing number of infectious diseases, and better designed environments reduce accidents. By contrast, no available treatment will modify the intellectual disability that accompanies Down's Syndrome. Thus, medical advances over the next decade are likely to increase the prevalence of the syndrome rather than reduce it.

The rise in prevalence of Down's Syndrome overshadows any reductions in the incidence of new cases that may have occurred. When one views the natural history of Down's Syndrome from conception onwards, this imbalance between incidence and prevalence appears even more of a paradox. The risk of spontaneous abortion with Down's Syndrome is about four times that of normal conceptions. In a sense one might consider that in the normal reproductive process the "natural" fate of a conception with this, and many other chromosomal anomalies, is embryonic death, and the "pathology" is survival through a normal gestation period and beyond. We estimate that of every 100 conceptions with the chromosomal anomaly of Down's Syndrome, only 23 survive to birth, and only 10 survive util the age of seven years. Whereas, of 100 normal conceptions, 85 survive at birth, and 82 until the age of seven.

Prevalence can be expected to increase until incidence and mortality reach a stable balance. If live births are considered as the starting cohort, one ceiling will be set by mortality, with a maximum prevalence the same as prevalence at birth. However, if conceptions are considered as the starting cohort, and if the high rate of attrition of the anomaly between conception and birth should be reduced, the maximum prevalence could be higher.

So if we are to talk seriously about primary prevention, we have to consider two strategies for prevention. In the face of rising prevalence two alternatives might be weighed—prevention of conception and intervention after conception.

PREVENTION OF CONCEPTION

A program of prevention of conception would have as its target women known to be a high risk in bearing a child with Down's Syndrome. Two vulnerable groups of mothers are known: one is identified by genetic transmission (having borne a child with Down's Syndrome), the other by maternal age.

The complete elimination of genetic transmission of Down's Syndrome would have virtually no effect on the incidence in the population (although that in no way diminishes the significance of prevention as it benefits individual families). The contribution of genetically transmitted forms to the incidence of Down's Syndrome is estimated at only 1.3%, and most cases will not be prevented until a case has occurred within a family.

The influence of maternal age on total incidence is much more striking. In New York City only 1.5% of mothers were over the age of 40, but they were likely to have contributed 16% of the cases of Down's Syndrome at birth, or ten times their proportionate share. The 7% of mothers 35 years and over were likely to have contributed 35% of the cases, or five times their proportionate share.

Thus, the incidence of Down's Syndrome would fall automatically if older women prevented conception. If this is considered desirable, the first step would be *education.* The hazard to offspring of older women should be made widely known. Some couples may prefer to risk having an infant with Down's Syndrome. Many others would undoubtedly choose to modify their fertility. It is, of course, their choice. However, couples should be given the knowledge that will allow them to make informed choices about childbearing. The argument might be advanced that to inform the public of the risk of a rare event would induce unnecessary anxiety. This argument is no more sound, with regard to older parents and Down's Syndrome, than it is with regard to smoking and lung cancer or fast motoring and traffic accidents. In the case of Down's Syndrome, an uninformed family can pay a high price indeed.

It is a principle of effective health education, however, that a health message which specifies a risk should also specify a solution, which, in this case, is *birth control.* Family planning and contraceptive advice should be fully available to older couples.

INTERVENTION AFTER CONCEPTION

It is likely that these methods would have some effect on incidence, but the effect would probably be slight. Many older women want to have children, and there are many sound family and social reasons for deferring childbearing to well into the thirties. It is also important to bear in mind that even if there were a large reduction in the fertility of older women, some two-thirds of the incidence of new cases of Down's Syndrome would remain untouched. At present, we estimate that in New York City two-thirds of infants with Down's Syndrome are born to women under 35 years of age.

It follows that if we want to achieve complete prevention we must consider intervention after conception. The available form of intervention is prenatal diagnostic screening. Amniocentesis makes this possible; abnormal fetuses can be identified during pregnancy and then, if the parents so desire, aborted.

As a problem of individual medicine, the prevention of Down's Syndrome has been made feasible by prenatal diagnosis and selective abortion. Indeed, many parents and doctors have already put these preventive measures into practice. In populations, too, the prenatal diagnosis and prevention of nearly all cases of Down's Syndrome are technically feasible, and it seems to us that they may become acceptable to many social groups as well. The key to transforming the diagnostic procedure from a clinical measure for sporadic use into a public health measure for systematic use is to adapt it as a screening device. A public health program based on the screening of many pregnant women requires that we evaluate the dangers of the procedures, the specificity and sensitivity of the tests, the risks to maternal health of induced abortions, the yield in terms of reduction of incidence, the costs and benefits to the community and, not least, the ethics of the program.

Should a prenatal diagnostic screening program be confined to the two known high-risk groups, i.e. those at genetic risk and older mothers? In the strategy of intervention there is no logical necessity, although there may be a practical one, for limiting the objective of a public health program to a partial solution. Almost total prevention of Down's Syndrome could be achieved by screening all pregnant women. In general, the ideology of public health endorses total prevention as a desirable objective. For a condition with rising prevalence like Down's Syndrome this objective is better achieved sooner than later.

A prenatal diagnostic screening program would be based on:

1. Amniocentesis.
2. Laboratory culture of aspirated cells for identification of karyotypes.
3. Induced abortion of affected fetus.
4. A comprehensive service to ensure that the population is covered in terms of information, access to screening, and obstetric services.
5. Evaluation of the program, in terms of efficacy and ethics.

1. *Amniocentesis*

Amniocentesis involves the aspiration of amniotic fluid from the uterine cavity. It is too soon to reach firm conclusions about the risks to the mother and the fetus from this procedure, but at present the evidence suggests that it is coming to be regarded as a minor surgical procedure. It seems unlikely to give rise to serious consequences if done under good conditions. More and better analyzed data are being collected and are urgently needed.

2. *Laboratory Screening*

The success rate of culture in experienced laboratories is now well above 90% of first attempts. The success rate per pregnancy, including repeat cultures, is about 95%.

Karyotyping for Down's Syndrome anomalies is now very reliable. The karyotype of trisomy 21 has proved specific for Down's Syndrome. No case with the karyotype in all the cells cultured has been without the phenotype. However, misdiagnosis could occur in two rare circumstances and reduce specificity to less than the apparent 100%. One is mosaicism, in which the cells of the fetus comprise both normal and trisomic types. If only abnormal cells were to be aspirated or cultured, a phenotypically normal or near normal fetus could be mistakenly aborted. The other is with twins dissimilar for Down's Syndrome, in which the presence of a normal twin might be missed if only anomalous cells were cultured.

The karyotyping is highly sensitive as well as specific. The known conditions that diminish this sensitivity are found in rare instances. With mosaicism, normal cells might be cultured and the child could prove to have phenotypic Down's Syndrome at birth, and the same applies to twins dissimilar for Down's Syndrome.

We conclude that the diagnosis of Down's Syndrome by karyotype, while not foolproof, is almost completely reliable, specific, and sensitive. The use of mass methods might reduce this precision if the extension to many laboratories is not made with the utmost attention to maintaining standards.

3. *Induced Abortion*

A screening program must offer termination to all those in whom the chromosomal anomaly is detected. The numbers needing abortion will be small compared to the total number of women now availing themselves of induced abortions where it is legal. In New York City for instance, the maximum increment would be 0.2% of the 70,000 abortions performed annually.

In weighing the risks and benefits we lay aside for the moment the critical question for any mother, which is whether she chooses to bear a child with the anomaly. We consider here only the secondary question of the medical procedures. Women selected for and electing abortion because of Down's Syndrome would tend to be older, and more advanced in pregnancy at the time of abortion, than others in whom abortion is induced. Although abortions in such women have a higher than average risk of complications, the appropriate comparison is with the outcome of uninterrupted pregnancies in women with similar characteristics. The raised morbidity and mortality associated with pregnancy and childbirth in older women are generally more serious than that associated with abortion, for instance, prolonged labor, forceps extraction, or caesarean section.

To summarize, neither the dangers of amniocentesis, the limitations of the diagnostic test, nor the risks of abortion in the few cases of Down's Syndrome which would be detected provide grounds for rejecting a public health program aimed at the elimination of Down's Syndrome.

4. *Comprehensive Service*

We now take up the question of the organization of such a program. Manpower is the first need. The small increment in induced abortions could easily be absorbed by existing services. But in order to carry out amniocentesis on women who elect to have it done, obstetricians will have to be recruited, trained, and persuaded of its value. Since the procedure is becoming part of regular obstetric services, the main problem will be the provision of service for all by those already skilled in giving it. A larger number of obstetricians and supporting staff will be required for a full program. However, although the scale of the undertaking would be large, it would not require a qualitative change in the structure of obstetric services which already carry out systematic prenatal screening for many conditions.

For laboratories too, the program would not be too difficult, although here the necessary skills are less common than on the obstetric side. More laboratory workers will have to be trained in cell culture and karyotyping.

Health education would be needed to ensure access and use and to keep the public informed of the dangers and benefits of the screening program.

Ongoing education. Public health agencies would also have to collect data and monitor the program. Sufficient routine data should be acquired to check the attributes of the participating population, diagnostic standards of specificity and sensitivity, rates of complications according to patient attributes, and expenditure.

There is ample room for technical development, both with amniocentesis and laboratory procedures. Amniocentesis early in pregnancy would provide a great advantage in a screening program. So would rapid and economical karyotyping. Computer methods for chromosomal typing are well advanced and may soon be adapted for routine operation. The demands of an active screening program are likely to stimulate such developments.

5. *Efficacy and Ethics*

The costs of a preventive program, when estimated from current fees for the procedures carried out on a sporadic basis for individuals, are high and direct economic benefits to public finances would be deferred for five years or more. The costs of the procedures carried out routinely on a mass scale would be much less, but still are likely to be high.

The cost of screening mothers over 30, at the current rates charged in New York City, would certainly be less than that of caring for the cases of Down's Syndrome among them. We are less certain about the balance of costs, at current rates, of screening the whole pregnant population. But is a detailed estimate of money costs required? The lifelong care of severely retarded persons is so burdensome in almost every human dimension that no preventive program is likely to outweigh the burden.

Although society has been tardy in wholeheartedly adopting even proven preventive measures as public policy, there is a precedent in mental retardation—namely, the screening and prevention of phenylketonuria (P.K.U.). The P.K.U. program in the United States is in some aspects less efficient than the program proposed for Down's Syndrome is likely to be. In Down's Syndrome the diagnostic test is more specific and more sensitive. The remedy is more certain and the expenditure of family and community resources in identified cases is less. P.K.U. prevention requires careful medical and family supervision of the affected child. From the point of view of efficacy, in reducing community prevalence, the total prevention of Down's Syndrome could reduce the prevalence of severe mental retardation by 25%. The total prevention of P.K.U. by current means will reduce the prevalence of severe mental retardation by only 1%.

In turning to ethics, we face the weightiest issues relating to the program. However, the ethical questions raised are no more difficult than those raised by any program that offers elective abortion, and in some important aspects they are less. There are three situations:

1. If elective abortion in normal pregnancy is acceptable, then the ethics of the Down's Syndrome program need no defense.
2. If induced abortions are acceptable in cases where the probability of fetal abnormality is high, as in rubella, or on the grounds of mental and social stress associated with the pregnancy, then again the ethics of the program need no defense. The element of specific selection introduced by a

preventive program for Down's Syndrome is no different from these cases.

3. If indeed abortion is never justified, or is justified only where the mother's life is at stake, then the program cannot be defended.

Individuals hold values covering all these contingencies, and the individual choice will always be made according to these values. Societies too, have legal and social policies that cover all these contingencies. New York State and Japan provide examples of the first type, where there are no bars to legal abortion. Britain and Sweden, where, again, there would be no legal bars to the proposed preventive program for Down's Syndrome, are examples of the second type. In some countries all abortions are illegal and can only be obtained by those rich or powerful enough to circumvent the law or to travel. Like abortion, the prevention of Down's Syndrome in such countries would be the privilege of the wealthy.

CONCLUSION

We have tried to touch on those issues which we felt might call for restraint in discussing, testing and perhaps mounting a preventive program for Down's Syndrome. On all counts, we conclude that a testing program is feasible and that it should be widely discussed and considered by those concerned with the future of Down's Syndrome. The testing program must take into account the need for experience and training in surgical and laboratory procedures; therefore, it should develop gradually and in stages. The phasing must also take into account the need for maintaining standards in all procedures and for their auditing and control.

We propose that in the first phase prenatal screening be offered to all pregnant women aged 40 years and over, in conformity with current individual practice in obstetrics. Since for older mothers the risk of bearing a child with Down's Syndrome is high, the yield of the screening will be high. On the other hand the risk of complications with abortion is greater than for younger women and the chances of a further pregnancy are reduced should they abort after amniocentesis. For these reasons, special care will have to be taken in the first phase and the results should provide a touchstone for expanding the program.

The numbers screened are built up by extending the target group in successive phases so that the risk of the procedure could be adequately evaluated in each phase and the community informed before the next stage is implemented. The program would require that every woman subjected to amniocentesis be followed at least until delivery. This is an ethical requirement and what is learned from it should enhance the informed quality of the consent given by participants in the screening procedure.

We cannot predict the proportion of women who would accept the offer of the screening test and an induced abortion, if it were positive. The rate of acceptance will be partly a measure of the vigor with which the program is explained and made accessible to the public.

We ventured into this evaluation tentatively. But we have completed it with a conviction that, where abortion laws permit, there is no need and no justification for delay in exploring the possibilities of a prenatal diagnostic screening program for Down's Syndrome. To effect the policy advocated here will bring relief to the community and a new assurance to prospective parents. These benefits are already available to a few, and more should be offered the choice.

REFERENCES

1. Stein, Z. and Susser, M.: HSMHA Hlth Rep., 86,650, 1971.
2. Stein, Z., Susser, M. and Guterman, A. V.: Screening programme for prevention of Down's Syndrome. *Lancet*, 305-310, 1973.
3. Tredgold, A. F. *Mental Deficiency*. London: William Wood & Co., 1:212, 2nd Edition, MDCCCCXIV, Survey of 1904, January, 1914.

7

Developmental Progress in Down's Syndrome

Jack B. Share, Ph.D.

How does one cope with such dramatic questions as, "What is my child's potential?" "Can he ever attend school?" "What is his optimal functioning?" These and other such questions are often put to the various professional people who come in contact with the families of Down's Syndrome (D.S.) children. They are often very difficult to answer. Yet, when there is a pattern of growth, then there is potential prediction. Optimal functioning can only be expected as a result of optimal development of capabilities.

Many problems that confront the parents of D.S. children seem to have developed from a lack of certainty as to what they can expect from their retarded child, and their subsequent failure to follow through with a positive program of training and education. For many years it was thought that the average D.S. child was unable to accomplish developmental landmarks, such as walking, talking, toilet training, etc., until well after his fifth birthday. It has now been well established that D.S. children are able to do many of these tasks much earlier than once thought. Furthermore, there appears to be a pattern of development among D.S. children, as among normal children, but at a slowed-down rate.

In an attempt to answer some of the questions and to reduce the accompanying anxieties about what to expect of a D.S. child, a longitudinal study documenting the growth and development of D.S.

children was carried out through the Child Development Clinic at the Los Angeles Childrens Hospital (1, 2, 3). Aspects of this investigation were selected and applied to a young D.S. population in New Zealand, as part of a cross-sectional investigation (4). Finally, a more recent study just completed reassessed a group of the Childrens Hospital longitudinal D.S. sample (N=76), whose ages now range from seven to 18 years. The present study sought to develop a wider base of information that would assist and enhance the early training, and the subsequent schooling, of these children, as well as to provide information for parents and professionals.

The Gesell developmental examination was utilized in the early assessments of the Down's Syndrome youngsters (6). It is of interest to note that infant tests owe their beginning to the developmental schedules proposed by Dr. Gesell in 1925 (7). Gesell attempted to establish developmental landmarks for the normal population. He further indicated that his method of developmental diagnosis was not limited to a measure of intelligence, but included all aspects related to the status of the nervous system, as expressed in four major areas: 1) motor coordination, 2) language development, 3) adaptive behavior, and 4) personal and social behavior.

Behavioral symptoms of maturity in all of these fields can be measured and recorded. Accordingly, Gesell described a series of normative schedules within these four areas in terms of normal expectancies for chronological ages of from one to seventy-two months.

In our study we selected landmarks from each of the four Gesell areas. They reflect areas of concern to many parents of D.S. children. The following tables present the median ages in months, age of onset of each landmark, and Gesell's normal population as compared to the median ages of the New Zealand D.S. population. The Los Angeles Childrens Hospital longitudinal sample is also included for comparison purposes. It will be noted in Table 1 that they are quite close in developmental landmarks to the New Zealand sample of children who were living at home.

It is also shown that the infant with D.S. follows a relatively normal motor pattern during the first six months of life. This, in part, accounts for the fact that many parents have difficulty accepting the

TABLE I

Motor Landmarks	Gesell Normals	Total	New Zealand Instit.	Home	Los Angeles Home
1. Holds head erect (zone II)	3	6	9	*5	3
2. Rolls over to prone	6	8	11	8	6
3. Sits unsupported for one minute erect	8	13	18	**12	11
4. Crawls & pivots	8	16	23	**15	13
5. Pulls to standing position	10	19	20	18	18
6. Creeps	10	18	19	18	17
7. Cruises at rail	12	21	23	20	—
8. Walks with support	13	22	26	*21	22
9. Stands unsupported	14	24	26	24	22
10. Walks unsupported	15	27	29	27	25
11. Walks upstairs with support	18	31	47	31	—
12. Seats self in chair	18	30	36	29	—
13. Walks downstairs with support	21	32	43	32	—
14. Goes up and down stairs alone	24	39	43	39	—

*p=.05 level of significance
**p=.02 level of significance

retardation based on early physical measures alone. However, from then on there is a gradual, but growing, discrepancy in the subsequent progress. By the time the infant reaches one year of age, he is often developmentally four to five months behind his chronological age. This lag nearly doubles by the time the child reaches his second birthday.

In Table 2, one can note that the area of slowest progress is in the acquisition of language. It is evident here that the normal infant is able to accomplish in ten months what frequently takes a child with Down's Syndrome nearly two years to master. This delay is maintained consistently throughout the other significant landmarks in the verbal area. In addition, it should be pointed out that, due to poor articulation, the speech of children with Down's Syndrome is often difficult to comprehend. On the other hand, their receptive language is remarkably better than their expressive ability. That is, D.S. children tend to be able to follow through on many commands,

TABLE 2

Language Landmarks	Gesell Normals	Total	New Zealand Instit.	Home	Los Angeles Home
1. Laughs aloud	4	7	10	6	5
2. Says "dada" and "mama"	10	15	13	16	24
3. Obeys simple commands (ball throwing - 2 directions)	18	29	32	29	41
4. Word combinations (2-3)	21	40	45	39	44
5. Sentences (3 words)	24	50	—	50	46

TABLE 3

Personal-Social Landmarks	Gesell Normals	Total	New Zealand Instit.	Home	Los Angeles Home
1. Smiles	2	4	6	3	3
2. Takes solids well	7	11	14	10	10
3. Feeds self in part	9	17	24	17	24
4. Drinks from cup unassisted	21	30	37	29	30
5. Feeds self "fully"	24	33	43	32	35
6. Urine control, daytime	24	34	33	34	39
7. Bowel control	24	36	41	35	34
8. Dresses self—simple garment	24	44	51	43	44
9. Dresses partially	36	50	—	50	66
10. Washes/dries hands and face	42	50	48	50	56
11. Brushes teeth unaided	48	48	—	48	58
12. Ties a knot (shoes)	60	—	—	—	—

attesting to the generally higher development in their receptive, as compared to their expressive, language.

The overall picture in Table 3 is similar to the pattern noted in the motor development in Table 1, in that up to six months of life fairly normal progress occurs. Thereafter, such tasks as feeding, dressing, and other self-care accomplishments are acquired very slowly. On the average they lag from ten to twenty-four months behind the normal population. It is revealing to find that the devel-

TABLE 4

Adaptive Landmarks	Gesell Normals	Total	New Zealand Instit.	Home	Los Angeles Home
1. Transfers objects in hands	7	11	13	11	—
2. Draws or imitates circle	24	48	64	47	—
3. Copies a cross	48	65	—	65	—
4. Copies a square	54	65	—	65	—

opmental discrepancies around such personal social habits as toilet training, bladder and bowel control are minor. These observations support the notion that children with Down's Syndrome can be trained in basic self-care functions, especially if certain repetitious patterns and set routines are followed. The three R's—Routine, Relaxation, and Repetition—helpful in teaching basic self-care to a young normal child, are also applicable to the Down's Syndrome child. Behavior shaping techniques, reverse chaining (doing steps in reverse), and token economy programs have greatly enhanced the establishment of basic personal-social skills.

In Table 4 we again notice the similar rate of progression as found in the motor and personal-social areas. The impact of institutionalization shows up dramatically here. The child institutionalized falls further and further behind. The negative aspects of institutionalization of young children have been well documented in the literature (8, 9, 10).

Motor development represented the area in which the Down's Syndrome children were most mature. The majority of these children are capable of walking, running, squatting, and climbing stairs. And they exhibit adequate motor coordination for the performance of simple tasks, such as stacking blocks and stringing beads, by five years of age. The majority of the children living at home were at least partially toilet-trained before three years of age. However, even those who were toilet-trained needed some help in the bathroom until six years of age.

Speech development represented the most limited area of development. None of the youngsters had speech qualitatively on par with the average child of his developmental age. Many of the mothers reported that although the children's attention span for assigned tasks was short, they could play for relatively long periods of time with things which they themselves had elected to do.

Their personalities varied—shy, bossy, modest, aggressive, passive, compliant, negativistic—in the same way that personalities of normal children vary. The majority seen were alert and responsive to their social environment.

A pertinent question now arises. What are some of the developmental characteristics which need to be taken into consideration in a modification, or presentation, of nursery or preschool material to young, moderately retarded or trainable Down's Syndrome children? When receptive and expressive language abilities were compared, the D.S. children were found to be similar to normal children in that their comprehension of language was better than their ability to use speech. Directions need to be simple and unequivocal. In the overall development of the normal child priority is placed on the acquisition of speech, after walking has been established (roughly that period of time after fifteen months of age). From then on, the vocabulary increases rapidly and words begin to be used in combination. With trainable D.S. children, the sequence is the same, but it is extremely delayed. The speech of D.S. children develops during the fourth, fifth, and sixth years of life with, of course, some exceptions. In other words, speech develops at the mental ages of fifteen months to two and a half or three years.

None of the youngsters seen could use words which denoted spatial relationships of even the simplest kinds, such as prepositions, "in," "on," "under," "on top of," etc. However, the more capable children were able to carry out instructions which involved the comprehension of such relationships. It is felt that with more repetition and demonstration on the part of parents, teachers, etc., many of these youngsters are capable of learning to carry out actions which involve some understanding of these elementary relations. This is an area in which D.S. children need to receive specific instructions, as opposed to average children who develop in this area through more or less casual observation.

It was possible to distinguish the relatively capable D.S. child more accurately by his purposeful and well-organized behavior than by his cooperativeness in the examining situation, or by the level of his speech development. The bright D.S. child whose speech lag was relatively great frequently had developed vivid methods of communicating with gestures, whereas the duller D.S. child with the same lag in speech had failed to devise any helpful substitute. On the basis of these observations, it would seem profitable to concentrate as early as possible on stimulating speech development with D.S. children, since speech inadequacy may be detrimental to future mental development as language becomes more and more essential to thinking.

It was further noted in testing that more repetition of directions was necessary than with normal children. This is essentially related to the problems of securing good attention—traditionally, one of the major problems in working with a retarded child. There were children who did not seem to understand the meaning of the expressions, "show me," or "point to." The impression was created that this uncertainty was related to a lack of experience with this kind of request, rather than with a lack of ability to comprehend. For the teacher this would indicate that these children need training in "direction expressions," to insure that they understand what is to be done, before they are expected to comply with the instructions that use these expressions. These discrepancies were most striking in the youngsters who were living in institutions.

In another finding we noted that if several objects were presented to a youngster, he often became confused and distracted by the presence of too many stimuli and needed to respond with some impulsive behavior before he could become organized to deal purposefully with the request. Another observation pointed to the advisability of allowing the child to look over the material long enough to become acquainted with it before requesting a particular activity of him. On the other hand it could be argued that this period of spontaneous exploration could lead to frustration. Here is a child trying to manipulate the material in a manner to which it does not lend itself, such as trying to put the square block in the round hole. But then, are not the child's manner of approach and his ability to cope with the material also a matter of interest to us?

The findings of the recently completed follow-up study of the Los Angeles Childrens Hospital D.S. longitudinal sample supported the reliability of the early Gesell measures for predictive purposes into the school years (5). The Gesell measures, under two years of age, can be used to predict later Stanford Binet IQ's, Wide Range Achievement scores, as well as Vineland Social Maturity scores, and may thus assist in future educational planning for young D.S. children.

The D.S. developmental landmarks* can be utilized best as a guideline of current status of D.S. children as a group, rather than as set or fixed stages of development. It may well be that the D.S. children who are raised in what may be termed an "optimal environment" might have a much earlier age of onset on all of these landmarks. Guidelines do not place limits on a given child but rather provide information that D.S. children can at least do some of the tasks presented by a certain age, thereby allowing the parent, educator, and physician to plan ahead and encourage further development along the next steps.

* *Developmental Landmarks for Children with Down's Syndrome* is in booklet form and is available through the author.

REFERENCES

1. Share, J., Webb, A., and Koch, R.: A preliminary investigation of the early developmental status of mongoloid infants, *Amer. J. Ment. Defic.*, 66:238, 1961.
2. Share, J., Koch, R., Webb, A., and Graliker, B.: The longitudinal development of infants and young children with Down's Syndrome (mongolism), *Amer. J. Ment. Def.*, 68:685, 1964.
3. Fishler, K., Share, J., and Koch, R.: Adaptation of Gesell developmental scales for evaluation of development in children with Down's Syndrome (mongolism), *Amer. J. Ment. Def.*, 68:642, 1964.
4. Share, J.: *Epidemiological and Developmental Study of Down's Syndrome (Mongolism) Children under Six Years of Age in New Zealand.* Unpublished doctoral thesis, Universidad Nacional Autonoma de Mexico (U.N.A.M.), 1971.
5. Share, J. and Landman, G.: *Down's Syndrome Longitudinal Study,* Tech. Report, SERP 1972, A-7, UCLA, pp. 91, Nov., 1972.

6. GESELL, A. and AMATRUDA, C.: *Developmental Diagnosis, Normal and Abnormal Child Development,* N.Y.: Paul B. Hoeber, 1939.
7. GESELL, A.: *The Mental Growth of the Pre-school Child,* New York: Macmillan, 1925.
8. BOWLBY, J. (editor.): *Maternal Care and Mental Health,* World Health Organization monograph, series No. 2, 1952.
9. SPITZ, R. A.: Hospitalism: an inquiry into the genesis of psychiatric conditions in early childhood, *Psychoanalytic Study of the Child,* 1:53, 1945.
10. FARRELL, M. J.: The adverse effects of early institutionalization of mentally subnormal children, *Amer. J. of Diseases of Children,* 9:278, 1956.

8

Mental Development in Mosaic Down's Syndrome as Compared with Trisomy 21

KAROL FISHLER, PH.D.

One of the major contributions in the study of Down's Syndrome came from the work of Lejeune and his co-workers (1) in cytogenetics. These studies reported chromosomal aberrations concerned with trisomy of the number 21 chromosome. In addition to this most common type of Down's Syndrome, a variety of unusual types of other chromosomal aberrations has been reported. The cases of translocation, mosaicism, XXYY, Klinefelter's and Turner's Syndromes are well described and identified by their unique cell complement. However, only in children with Down's Syndrome has mental development been studied extensively by numerous examiners (2, 3, 4, 5). Some of these examiners report that many of their subjects showed only "partial" conditions of Down's Syndrome in their physical, mental or social aspects. These "atypical" characteristics were often at variance with the customary stereotype of a passive, affectionate personality with moderate to severe level of retardation of intellectual function.

It has been shown rather well that children with Down's Syndrome follow a unique pattern of development which approximates a normal distribution curve, but at a slower rate of progress. It is the deficit in the developmental and subsequently in the intellectual

FIGURE 1

DISTRIBUTION OF DQ AND IQ SCORES IN DOWN'S SYNDROME GROUP

N = 28

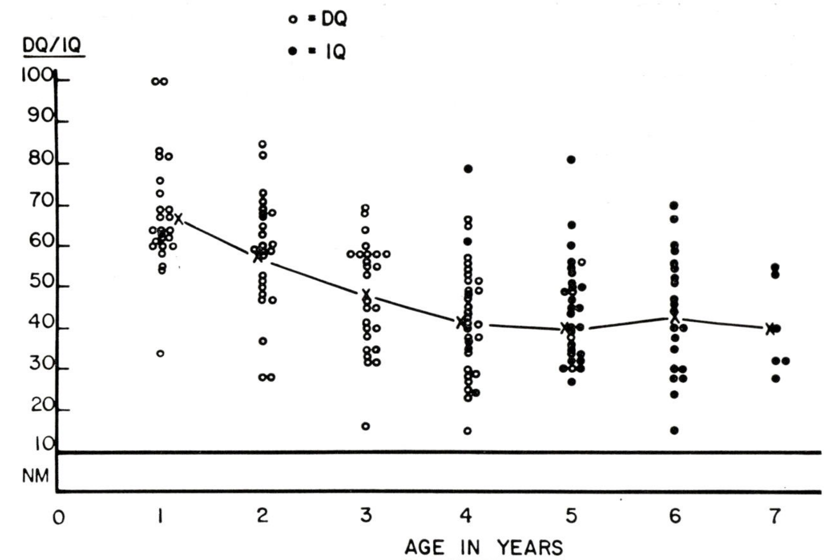

CORREL.COEFF.	r=.50	r=.64	r=.85	r=.82
PROBABILITY	p<.01	p<.01	p<.01	p<.01

achievements which is nearly universally present in this population.

Our own longitudinal study of developmental and mental growth in a Down's Syndrome group (6) showed what may be considered a "typical" developmental curve. The usual pattern of motor development suggests an increasing discrepancy between the gains made by normal children and by Down's Syndrome children after the first six months of life. A similar pattern of progress is also noted in the area of personal-social behavior, dealing with such accomplishments as feeding, dressing and toilet training. The area of slowest progress is language development, in which the Down's Syndrome group often lags significantly in comparison to normal children.

The "classical" distribution of DQ and IQ scores in a Down's Syndrome population is shown in Figure 1. It is immediately apparent that there is a tendency to score higher during the first and second years of life when using the Gesell Developmental Scales. There is a gradual decrease in DQ to a relative plateau at the age of three and four years. In fact, the scores on developmental tests at those age levels appear to be reliable predictors of the child's subsequent intellectual functioning. The level of intellectual achievement of older persons usually scatters from 30 to 50 IQ points.

We have psychometric studies on nearly 300 subjects with Down's Syndrome whom we have followed over the course of 10 to 15 years since our original study was conducted. Most of the subjects were seen for repeated psychometric testing, with some for as many as six, seven and nine annual evaluations. The developmental and intellectual progress on 255 subjects with 21 trisomy Down's Syndrome is shown in Figure 2.

The similarity of the two curves becomes almost immediately evident when comparing the findings with our initial impressions nearly ten years ago. It will be noted that young infants at the age of one year tend to score highest and then their score drops an average of 10 points in the second year of life. This trend is still much in evidence by the age of three years, at which point the development curve tends to plateau and remains fairly stable through the consecutive years of mental growth. These data fully confirm our earlier results and denote the customary leveling off process in the area of intellectual development by the age of four to five years, with the expected scatter from 30 to 50 IQ points.

DEVELOPMENTAL PROGRESS IN MOSAIC DOWN'S SYNDROME

Although some of the investigators recognize that certain individuals tend to achieve higher intellectual levels, it has been generally agreed that this ability is particularly true of mosaic Down's Syndrome. Clarke et al. (2) and Hamerton et al. (7) have reported two cases of normal intelligence in mosaic Down's Syndrome individuals.

FIGURE 2

DISTRIBUTION OF DQ AND IQ SCORES IN DOWN'S SYNDROME TRISOMY 21

N = 255

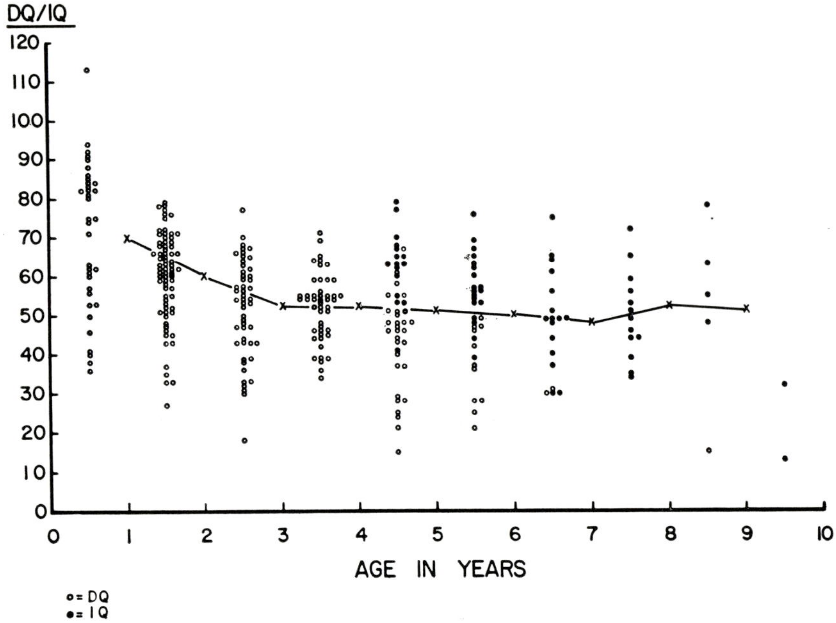

Other investigators (4, 8, 9, 10) describe their cases as of average or "normal" intelligence. Of special interest is the notion of Polani (11), who feels that a discrepancy between somatic characteristics of Down's Syndrome and relatively good intellectual functioning appears to be an "index of potential mosaicism." One may further speculate a possible relationship between the complement of aberrant cells in mosaicism to intellectual development.

DESCRIPTION OF SAMPLE GROUP OF CHILDREN WITH MOSAIC DOWN'S SYNDROME

The sample of 15 children with mosaic Down's Syndrome, on which this report is based, is made up of eight males and seven

FIGURE 3

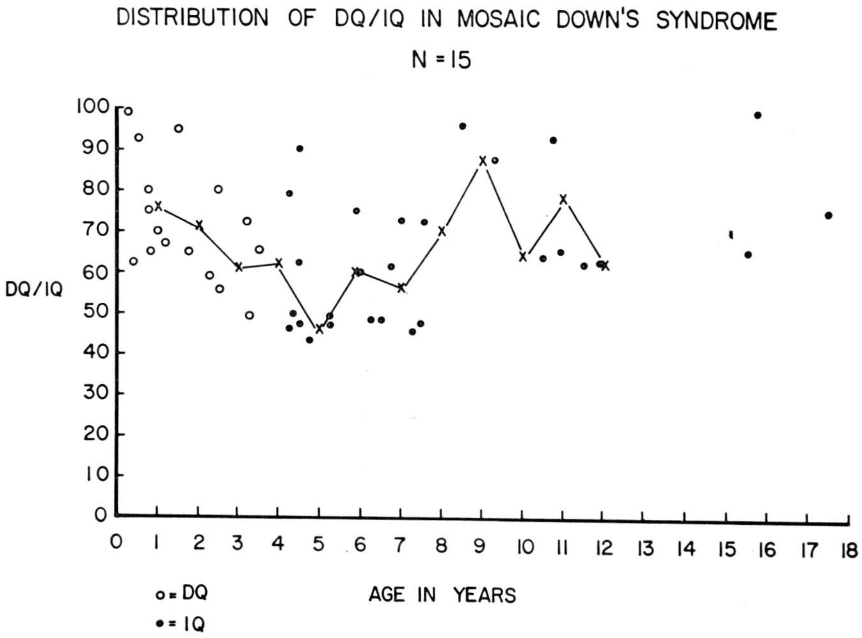

females, with a wide range of age, from four to more than 18 years of age. Similarly, the age of referral for study ranged from 12 days of age up to 15½ years. Six of our patients were seen for the first time at less than one year level, and the longest follow-up is in excess of ten years with one family. It should be pointed out that each child was seen for several psychometric evaluations, with only two children seen twice. Among all of the children of school age, only one attended a regular grade class in a public school system, while all others were enrolled in the special education programs or kindergarten. All of the preschool youngsters are at home and doing well, with one or two children being considered for a nursery class experience. One child, a girl of 6½ years, was killed several years ago in an auto accident. She is not included in this sample.

TABLE I

Comparison of IQ Levels Between Mosaic and Trisomy 21 Down's Syndrome Subjects Matched for Age and Sex

	MOSAIC			TRISOMY 21	
No.	Age	IQ	Sex	Age	IQ
1	18-3	73	F	18-9	71
2	16-2	89	M	16-0	71
3	13-1	81	F	13-1	70
4	12-10	59	M	12-6	55
5	12-4	71	M	12-6	18
6	12-3	65	M	12-5	31
7	10-7	55	F	10-7	60
8	9-8	63	F	9-11	55
9	9-6	87	M	9-7	59
10	8-3	58	F	8-1	51
11	7-9	59	F	7-9	53
12	7-5	75	M	7-0	47
13	5-1	57	M	5-2	44
14	4-8	76	M	5-0	75
15	4-0	43	F	4-0	46
Mean:	10-1	67		10-1	53
S.D.		12.9			15.7
Range:		43-89			18-75

$t = 2.64$
$p < 0.01$

Results

The distribution of developmental achievements in terms of DQ scores and subsequent assessments of mental potential in terms of IQ scores is reported in Figure 3. It should be pointed out that, whereas the range of initial test results scattered from 59 to 100, with a mean score of 74, the most recent test scores ranged from 43 to 89, with a mean score of 67. This mean value for the entire sample compares closely with the mean IQ of 65 for the 20 cases of mosaicism reported by Rosecrans (12).

It will be noted that the developmental curve drawn for the mosaic Down's Syndrome does not follow any set trend as the one for the trisomy 21 group. There is little doubt though that the individuals in the mosaic group manifest considerably higher intellectual potential. Table 1 shows a comparison of IQ levels between mosaic and trisomy 21 Down's Syndrome subjects, who were carefully matched for age and sex. The obtained value of $t=2.64$ is significant at better than $p<0.01$ level.

This finding indicates the need for caution on the part of physicians and other professional personnel involved in the care of very young children with Down's Syndrome in recommending early placement outside of the home. The variability of mental potential in Down's Syndrome is a good reason for avoiding institutionalization in early infancy. It is now well established that institutionalization generally decreases the opportunity to develop maximal potential.

Discussion

In attempting to analyze some of the best achievements which the mosaic Down's Syndrome group demonstrated on psychological tests, it was noted that those individuals with the higher IQ levels often demonstrated an unusually good quality of speech. In contrast to the usual flat, hoarse, and frequently unclear quality of the speech of the typical child with Down's Syndrome, some of these subjects had well-modulated speech and normal intonation. Similarly, they generally manifested better vocabulary, comprehension and ability to deal with numerical concepts. A good example of a child who consistently maintained positive gains over the course of many years is shown in Figure 4.

Although most of the trisomy 21 Down's Syndrome subjects manifested some visual-perceptual deficit, as evidenced in their poor ability to handle paper and pencil tasks, several of the mosaic group individuals were able to reproduce various geometric forms quite well (see Figures 5, 6 and 7). These findings suggest that those subjects who show a greater degree of distortions in their drawings often experience a distinct learning disorder in academic pursuits, notably reading, writing or arithmetic. Furthermore, it appears that the occurrence of these difficulties is more likely in those individuals with lower IQ levels. If it is true that tests such as Bender-Gestalt identify significant deficit in this area which is also typical of other children with organic dysfunction, one might speculate that "brain damage" patterns would be more typical of the group.

FIGURE 4

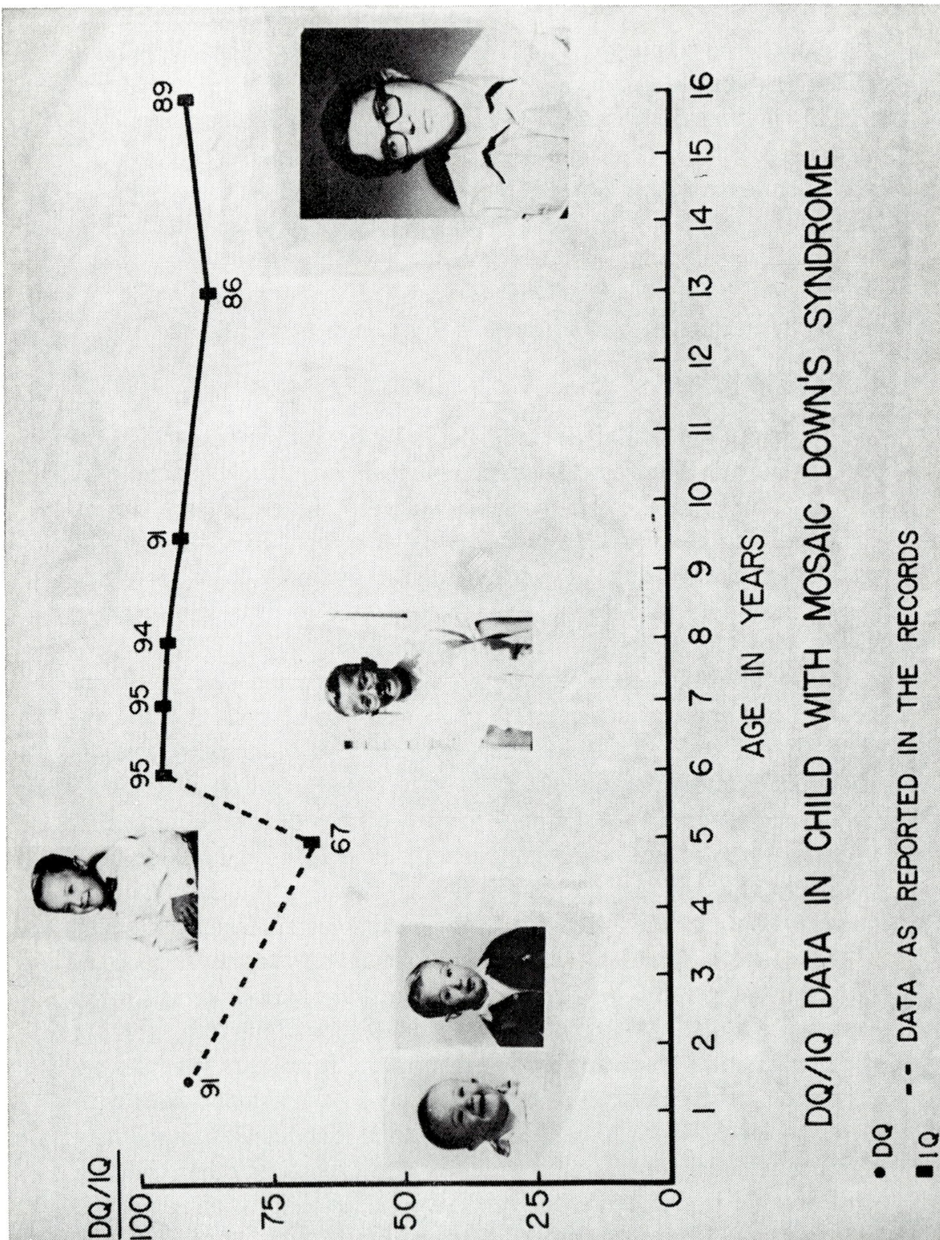
DQ/IQ
100
75
50
25
0
91
67
95
95
94
91
86
89
1 2 3 4 5 6 7 8 9 10 11 12 13 14 15 16
AGE IN YEARS
DQ/IQ DATA IN CHILD WITH MOSAIC DOWN'S SYNDROME
• DQ
■ IQ
-- DATA AS REPORTED IN THE RECORDS

FIGURE 5

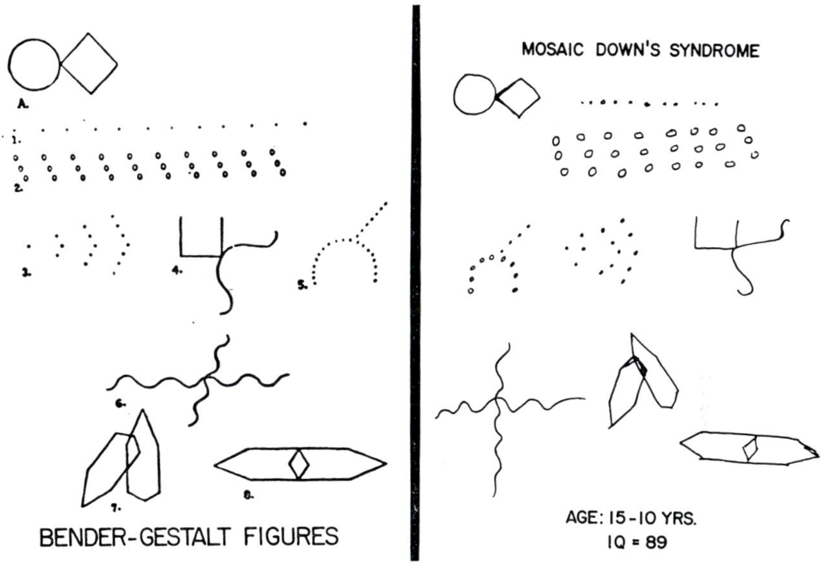

FIGURE 6

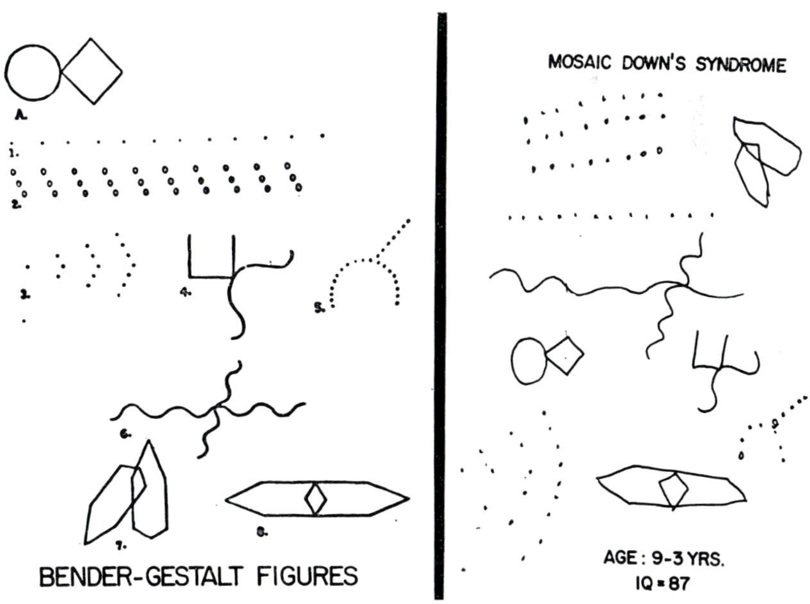

FIGURE 7

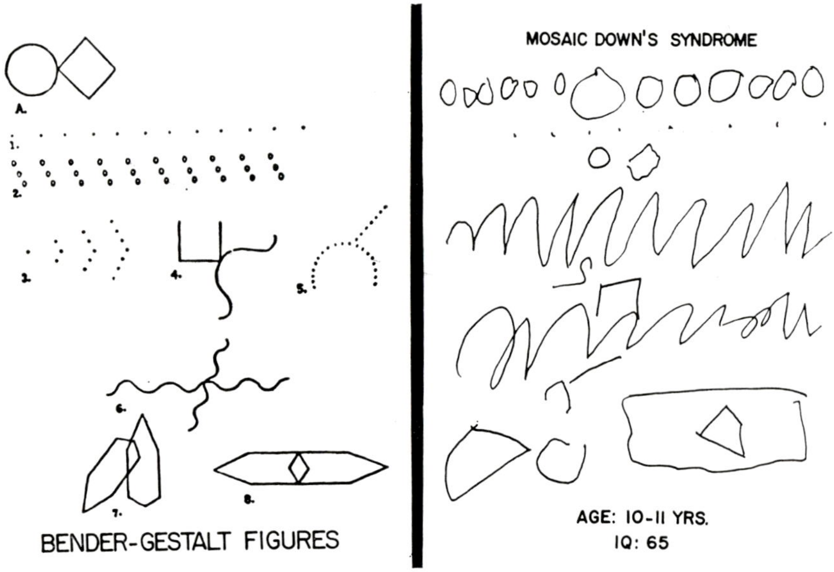

As for the question of the amount of chromosomal materials being directly related to the degree of defects, our present techniques do not permit such a conclusion. One wonders if the percentage of abnormal cells of the mosaic Down's Syndrome individuals correlates with their intellectual status and physical stigmata. Domino and Newman (13) were unable to show any relationship between physical stigmata of the 21 trisomy and intellectual development, although another investigator (11) feels that less evidence of physical signs and relatively good intellectual functioning provide an "index of potential mosaicism." Our own data on 15 mosaic Down's Syndrome subjects, in terms of their complement of the normal cell percentage, is shown in Table 2, and does not permit any clear conclusions.

From the behavioral point of view, most of our mosaic Down's Syndrome subjects did not vary from the trisomy 21 group. They seemed to be sociable and, for the most part, friendly in interpersonal contacts, but generally tended to perform better in a one-to-one situa-

TABLE 2

Comparison of IQ Levels with Percentage of Normal Cells in Mosaic Down's Syndrome
N=15

No.	Sex	Age	IQ	% Normal Cells*
1	F	18-3	73	93
2	M	16-2	89	53
3	F	13-1	81	65
4	M	12-10	59	81
5	M	12-4	71	54
6	M	12-3	65	27
7	F	10-7	55	36
8	F	9-8	63	11
9	M	9-6	87	54
10	F	8-3	58	78
11	F	7-9	59	81
12	M	7-5	75	85
13	M	5-1	57	72
14	M	4-8	76	39
15	F	4-0	43	33

* Formula for calculation % Normal cells= $\frac{46}{46+47} \times 100$

tion. A fair number though, particularly those with lower mental potential, would become more easily frustrated and distracted when under pressure.

CONCLUSIONS

The observations and serial assessments of mental status in 15 subjects with mosaic Down's Syndrome support most earlier reports in the literature that these individuals often tend to achieve higher intellectual levels than typical children with trisomy 21. In our experience with 15 mosaics some developed better verbal facility and less visual-perceptual difficulties (which interfere with learning ability) than anticipated for a typical Down's Syndrome population. Their behavioral adjustment and personality characteristics are not in variance with similar characteristics in other types of Down's Syndrome, and are more likely reflective of one's own home situation. The present technique of chromosome analysis does not, as yet, permit valid conclusions about the complement of abnormal cells and intellectual status in mosaicism. From the practical point of view, it is felt that any child with Down's Syndrome who scores an IQ higher than 55 upon reaching the age of four to five years, and whose speech is relatively normal, can be viewed as a suspected case of mosaicism. A chromosomal analysis done concurrently with serial assessments of mental status is the best indicator in verifying or disproving such suspicions.

REFERENCES

1. LEJEUNE, J., GAUTHIER, M., and TURPIN, R.: Les chromosomes humains en culture de tissus. *Compt. rend Acad. d. sc.*, 1959, 248, 602.
2. CLARKE, C. M., EDWARDS, J. H. and SMALLPIECE, V.: 21-Trisomy/normal mosaicism in intelligent child with some mongoloid characters. *Lancet*, 1961, 1, 1028-30.
3. HAYASHI, T., HSU, T. C. and CHAO, D.: A case of mosaicism in mongolism. *Lancet*, 1962, 1, 218.
4. LINDSTEN, J., ALVIN, A., GUSTAVSON, K. H. and FRACCARO, M.: Chromosomal mosaicism in a girl with some features of mongolism. *Cytogenetics*, 1962, 1, 20.
5. FINLEY, W. H., FINLEY, S. C., ROSECRANS, C. J. and TUCKER, C. C.: Normal/21-trisomy mosaicism. *Amer. J. Diseases Child.*, 1966, 112, 144.
6. FISHLER, K., SHARE, J. and KOCH, R.: Adaptation of Gesell developmental scales for evaluation of development in children with Down's Syndrome (mongolism). *Am. J. Ment. Def.*, 1964, 68, 642.
7. HAMERTON, J. L., GIANELLI, F., and POLANI, P. E.: Cytogenetics of Down's Syndrome (mongolism): 1: Data on a consecutive series of patients referred for genetics counseling and diagnosis. *Cytogenetics*, 1965, 4, 171.
8. WEINSTEIN, E. D., and WARKANY, J.: Maternal mosaicism and Down's Syndrome (mongolism). *J. Pediat.*, 1963, 63, 599.
9. VERRESEN, H., VAN DEN BERGHE, H., and CREEMERS, J.: Mosaic trisomy in phenotypically normal mother of mongol. *Lancet*, 1964, 1, 526.
10. RIDLER, M. A., SHAPIRO, A., and DELHANTY, J. D.: A mosaic mongol with normal leucocyte chromosomes. *Brit. J. Psychiat.*, 1965, 11, 183.
11. POLANI, P. E.: Cytogenetics of Down's Syndrome. In: Symposium on genetics. L. I. Gardner (ed.) *Ped. Clinics N. Amer.*, 1963, 10, 423.
12. ROSECRANS, C. J.: The relationship of normal/21-trisomy mosaicism and intellectual development. *Am. J. Ment. Def.*, 1968, 72, 562.
13. DOMINO, G., and NEWMAN, D.: Relationship of physical stigmata to intellectual subnormality in mongoloids. *Am. J. Ment. Def.*, 1965, 70, 541.

9

Present Approaches to Therapy in Down's Syndrome

GEORGE F. SMITH, M.D.

This report will discuss treatment in its broadest sense, so it will be necessary to comment upon the medical, educational and social changes which are of importance in the treatment of Down's Syndrome. Rather than being a proponent of any special form of treatment, it is important to discuss those factors inherent in Down's Syndrome which make the evaluation of any treatment program difficult. And I would like to present a recommendation for a program which would permit a more sensible evaluation of future therapeutic programs for the individual with Down's Syndrome.

In its simplest form, a therapeutic program in some way has to improve the patient's condition, make it worse or have no effect on it. Predicated on this concept is the knowledge that we know in advance what the individual or individuals would have been like if no intervention had taken place.

The crux of the problem in Down's Syndrome for the evaluation of therapeutic programs is the marked variability of physical, motor and mental abilities that exists within this group of individuals. While there are stereotypes by which we describe their physical and mental characteristics, the variability for any of these stereotyped features can be quite significant in a given individual.

Because of the variability of the physical features, there has always been an element of uncertainty in the diagnosis. This is particu-

TABLE I

Frequencies of Physical Signs in Mongolism Expressed as Percentages

Sign	Oster (1953) Children or adults	Levinson et al. (1955) Children or adults	Hall (1964) Newly born
Mouth:			
Habitually open	67	62	—
Fissured lips	—	56	—
*Small teeth	71	56	—
Irregular alignment	71	68	—
Large tongue	57	30	—
Protruding tongue	49	32	68
*Furrowed tongue	59	44	—
*Seemingly high-arched palate	67	74	—
Eyes:			
*†Oblique palpebral fissures	75	88	80
*Epicanthic folds	28	50	—
Speckled iris	70	30	42
Strabismus	23	14	—
Nystagmus	12	14	—
Ears:			
Prominent	47	50	—
Malformed	49	48	—
Small or absent lobes	82	80	57
Folded helix	—	—	53
†Dysplastic	—	—	62
Neck:			
Broad and short	39	50	—
†Abundant skin	—	—	81
Abdomen:			
Diastasis recti	—	76	—
Umbilical hernia	—	4	—
Genitalia:			
Small penis	98	50	—
Cryptorchism	27	20	—
Small scrotum	—	42	—
Head:			
*Flat occiput	74	82	—
Round shape	—	—	77
†Flat facial profile	—	—	89
Flat nasal bridge	59	62	79
Open fontanelle (after the age of 6 months)	—	16	—

TABLE I - *continued*

	Oster (1953) Children or adults	Levinson et al. (1955) Children or adults	Hall (1964) Newly born
Chest:			
Funnel type	5	12	—
Pigeon breasted	5	14	—
Flat nipples	—	56	—
Dorsolumbar kyphosis	—	14	—
Hands:			
*Short broad hands	69	74	—
Short fingers	—	70	—
Short 5th finger	57	66	—
*Curved 5th finger	48	68	32
One flexion crease on 5th finger	31	10	14
*†Four-finger crease	43	48	54
†Dysplastic middle phalanx 5th finger	—	—	58
Feet:			
Excessive space between 1 and 2 toes	47	44	46
Plantar furrow	—	28	—
Joints and Muscles:			
*†Hyperextensibility or hyperflexibility	47	—	77
Hyperabduction of hip joints	—	—	84
†Muscular hypotonia	21	—	77
Weak patella reflexes	—	—	84
†Dysplastic pelvis	—	—	67
†Lack of Moro reflex	—	—	82

*Ten most characteristic signs selected by Oster (1953).
†Ten best diagnostic signs in newly born (Hall 1964).

larly true for those physicians having had relatively little experience with the condition. Since 1959, with the advent of chromosome analysis, a correct diagnosis is now possible in every case. However, with the use of chromosome analysis, we have come to understand how deceptive the physical and mental characteristics can be in certain Down's Syndrome individuals.

VARIATIONS IN CLINICAL FINDINGS

Some of the more useful diagnostic physical features of Down's Syndrome, selected from the reports of Oster (15), Levinson et al. (12), and Hall (7), are seen in Tables 1 and 2. There is a fair agreement between the data of Oster and Levinson et al. in the percentage of child and adult Down's Syndrome individuals having characteristic physical features. However, for certain of the individual features, such as epicanthic folds and speckled iris, there is a marked difference in the frequencies in the two studies. In addition, all three studies show that the frequency of some of the physical manifestations occurs at a low rate in the Down's Syndrome population and that no one physical finding occurred in all of these individuals. The significance of these traits, for therapy evaluation purposes, is somewhat limited by the fact that they are not clearly definable and depend upon clinical impressions. As seen from the data of Hall, who worked with newborns, many of the traits are age dependent.

There is also a wide variation at the age at which these individuals progress through various stages of development. As can be seen in Table 3, a mean age for developmental stages can be established but there is an extremely wide range at which these stages are reached for any given Down's Syndrome child.

A biochemical evaluation of Down's Syndrome (17) also shows the marked variation in the values obtained for any given test. In general, for any given biochemical test, it is possible to obtain mean and standard deviation values different from the normal population. However, many of the values obtained for Down's Syndrome individuals will overlap those of the normal population so that there is no biochemical test that clearly differentiates the individual with Down's Syndrome from the normal population. In addition to this,

TABLE 2

Comparative Frequencies of Ten Critical Signs in the Newly Born. (Hall 1964)

Character	Mongols	Controls
Oblique palpebral fissures	46/57	2/86
Dysplastic ears	23/37	2/40
Excessive skin on back of neck	46/57	1/86
Flattened features	50/56	1/85
Four-finger palmar crease (either hand)	30/56	8/86
Dysplastic middle phalanx on digit V (either hand)	25/43	2/37
Hyperflexibility	43/56	14/86
Muscular hypotonia	43/56	3/86
Dysplastic pelvis	25/37	—/—
Absence of Moro reflex	44/54	6/85

TABLE 3

Mean Ages and Age Ranges at which Mongols Reached the Following Stages of Development

(After Erbs & Smith, 17*)

Event	Mean age in months	Range in months
Rolled over	7.7	1-36
Sat up	13.0	6-30
Stood (without support)	21.8	9-48
Walked	26.8	16-48
Bladder trained	35.2	24-48
Bowel trained	40.5	25-54

*See Chapter by Erbs and Smith in *Down's Anomaly,* p. 56, (17). Unpublished Observations—1962.

some of the abnormal biochemical findings also appear to be age dependent (18).

In situations where there is general agreement about an abnormal chemical finding in Down's Syndrome, controversy usually exists about its cause and interpretation. For example, the chemistry of a disease like phenylketonuria, caused by a homozygous pair of abnormal genes, can be fairly well understood, but a more complex situation is encountered in a disease like Down's Syndrome, which is caused by trisomy.

Data on intelligence also present us with certain difficulties when trying to evaluate treatment programs. All would agree that the largest group with Down's Syndrome falls into the IQ range of 25-49 (17). Much of this type of information depends heavily on the Stanford-Binet intelligence scale which may not be the best way to evaluate changes in response to therapy.

If one is to intervene using medical or educational treatment it is the young Down's Syndrome individuals, under the age of three years, who will probably show the most favorable response. However, it is also in this age group that we see the greatest variability in the Developmental Quotient (DQ) scores. For a small group of children under the age of three years, 23 percent had a DQ over 70, while 47 percent had a DQ between 50-69, and for 30 percent it was between 25-49 (13). For Down's Syndrome infants under one year of age, the figures are more dramatically in favor of high DQ scores, with between one-third and one-half of all infants having a DQ over 70 (11, 13, 15).

The difficulty arises in how to interpret these data when evaluating the effects of medical and educational treatment plans for young Down's Syndrome infants. The problem is compounded by the lack of information from longitudinal studies of intelligence levels. The study of Koch, Share, Webb and Graliker in 1963 (10) would indicate that there is a fairly high correlation coefficient (0.78) between the DQ at 14-24 months and the Stanford-Binet IQ at five years of age. It would seem, however, that more information is needed about the predictive value of the DQ scores and whether or not they are best correlated at a later age with the Stanford-Binet when evaluating treatment programs for Down's Syndrome children.

The aforementioned remarks on the clinical variation in Down's Syndrome do not include the marked differences that can be found in Down's Syndrome mosaics, which have to be considered when evaluating treatment results.

MEDICAL TREATMENT

Most therapies used in the treatment of Down's Syndrome have not lived up to their initial claims, when put to the test of scientific investigation. Others, about which beneficial claims have been made, have not yet been subjected satisfactorily to controlled investigation, so unbiased evaluation is not possible. Indeed, correct evaluation of drug therapy presents many problems and pitfalls for the investigator. Mental improvement is a frequently used standard for measuring a Down's Syndrome individual's response, which may be done either by looking for changes in DQ, IQ, or SQ (Social Quotient). These individuals are highly responsive to their environments so that small changes in test scores could be accounted for by added stimulation or merely new developmental changes associated with maturation. In addition, it is not certain that IQ and SQ tests are the best means of evaluating responses to therapy. There is as yet no form of medical treatment which has been proven to have significant merit.

The earliest form of therapy to be widely used was the administration of dessicated thyroid gland. This evolved naturally because Down's Syndrome individuals were initially classified as cretins, until their condition was recognized as a separate clinical entity. The efficacy of thyroid therapy has not been substantiated by clinical research (11) except in a small number of patients who have intercurrent hypothyroidism (2). Pituitary extract has been claimed to have a beneficial effect (2); however, this claim was not supported in the results of studies conducted by Berg, Kirman, Stern, and Mittwoch (3). Other drugs, such as thymus extract and glutamic acid, have been fashionable in the treatment of the mentally retarded and they were tried without success on Down's Syndrome individuals. It was suggested (14) that by using dehydroepiandrosterone the facies and the neuromuscular performance of individuals with Down's Syndrome could be improved. Controlled studies testing this claim did not validate it (6). Many unusual combinations of drugs and vitamins were proposed by Turkel (19). However, they were used without success in studies conducted by Bumbalo, Morelewicz, and Berens (4). A form of treatment which employs cellular extracts (Siccacell) and a vitamin-mineral-hormonal preparation has been proposed by Haubold, Loew, and Haefele-Niemann (8). However, the claim that this therapy produces improvement has been refuted by Bardon (1). White and Kaplitz (20) evaluated the vitamin-mineral-hormonal preparation without the addition of Siccacell and noted that the patients did no better than the controls.

Intensive physiotherapy with a regression to basic developmental patterns has been recommended for children with Down's Syndrome. This type of treatment has not been subjected to proper controlled investigation so that an informative evaluation of the effect cannot be made. However, in the ten or more years that these programs have been used, there is no evidence that there is a sustained beneficial effect for these individuals.

During the past ten to 15 years, parents of Down's Syndrome children have been inundated with supposedly scientific reports from the Detroit area on the use of combined drugs and vitamins. These reports are not from a scientific journal but are in the form of a booklet produced by a physician. This type of information has only served to confuse these parents. The scientific value of these reports for evaluating the effect of this type of therapy is worthless.

The most recent form of medical therapy has been the use of 5-hydroxytryptophan which will be commented on by two of the speakers at this conference. For my part, it is sufficient to say that Dr. Coleman's evaluation of this material was conducted in such a way that adequate conclusions could be reached.

Even though a specific form of medical therapy is not presently available in Down's Syndrome, good medical care has succeeded in keeping these individuals healthy and more productive. With the advent of antibiotics, corrective surgery, and good nutrition they can be maintained in a relative state of good health. The improved health has allowed these individuals to participate in educational and recreational programs and to do some forms of occupational activities, when available, as adults. The life expectancy for Down's Syndrome individuals in 1929 was nine years (16), by 1947 it had increased to 12 years, and for the years 1948 to 1957 it had increased to 18.3

years (5). The life expectancy has continued to improve and at the present time we are seeing Down's Syndrome individuals survive to the fifth, sixth, and seventh decades of life.

EDUCATIONAL TREATMENT

During the past ten years, it has been shown that much can be done to aid the Down's Syndrome individual to become a more useful person through special educational programs and occupational training. While many of these programs are new in this country, the concepts upon which they are based are old and were even recommended by Down and his successors at Earlswood, as can be inferred from the case records from 1858 onwards.

Special education enables these individuals to participate in a stimulating environment and helps to raise their abilities to the maximum level even though, by normal standards, this level is limited. Exploratory methods for teaching the subnormal are producing new information which can be applied to subsequent training programs.

Educational programs have now reached a level where they have to be judged by the same scientific techniques as apply to other forms of therapy. It is insufficient, in this day, to say that any form of educational program is adequate for the child with Down's Syndrome. If we are to know what form of education is most suitable for these individuals, the educators will have to give recognition to the variables in the physical and mental abilities and disabilities that exist in this syndrome, in order to properly evaluate their programs. These are the same variables that have plagued the physician in his evaluation of specific medical treatment programs.

Possibly one of the deficiencies in the educational programs is an inadequate definition of the purpose for which these children are being educated. In too many schools the purpose seems to be merely an exercise for the teacher so that he or she can complete statistical forms which are all important to the city or county board of education. Now that the Down's Syndrome individual is surviving into the later decades of life, the educators will need to have a more global view of these individuals and not limit their expectations to the years six through 18.

One of the criteria for being considered socially useful is to be productive. Within their limitations, Down's Syndrome individuals can perform a variety of useful and, at times, complicated tasks. There are many scientific questions that the educators will have to answer. For example, what educational techniques are most applicable in training these individuals to be productive in adult life? At what age is it possible to tell which child will benefit the most from an intensive educational experience, and at what age is the educational experience most beneficial?

Our ability to evaluate the potentials of these individuals may have to be examined in more specific ways. The Stanford-Binet test, while suitable for normal children, seems to be an unreliable predictor for too many children with Down's Syndrome. An example is provided by the book written by a Down's Syndrome patient in London, *The World of Nigel Hunt* (9). Nigel's score on the Stanford-Binet was in the 45 range, a range common for many Down's Syndrome individuals and one usually not associated with the ability to write a book.

The evaluation of any new educational programs will have to take into consideration the environmental and social changes that are rapidly occurring in the families of Down's Syndrome individuals, and in the communities in which they live. Increasingly favorable family attitudes towards the Down's Syndrome individual, which encourage parents and siblings to treat the Down's Syndrome child as just another family member, have given these individuals a new self-identity and self-assurance. Similar favorable social changes are occurring in most communities which are opening up new avenues of social participation. These and other similar factors could have a marked stimulating and gratifying effect on individuals with Down's Syndrome. Unless educators are conscious of the evolutionary environmental changes that are taking place outside of school, including improved health standards, they may overestimate the part their own educational techniques are playing in any improvement shown in these individuals. This type of overestimation on the part of the educator would have a bad effect in general since there would be a tendency to slow down the development of new specialized teaching programs for Down's Syndrome children.

NATIONAL TREATMENT PROGRAM

One gets the impression that the evaluation of medical or educational treatment programs for individuals with Down's Syndrome is today where the evaluation of treatment programs was ten years ago for children with leukemia. At that time independent groups were attempting to evaluate treatment programs on small numbers of children. Not only was it difficult to draw conclusions on small numbers but there was a large number of independent variables, such as the type of leukemia, age of onset, bias of the individual investigator, etc., which made data comparisons difficult and precluded the formation of any definite conclusions. However, once a national plan was organized for leukemia and special treatment centers established, data collection became easy and positive conclusions were reached. In the past decade the leukemia program for children has produced fantastic results and has been ahead of most other programs of cancer therapy.

Until a similar type of national unified program is established for evaluating medical and educational treatment programs for Down's Syndrome individuals, progress in this field will continue at an extremely slow rate. In a disease process which is plagued by so many variables, it is almost impossible for one professional or a group of professionals to get a large enough sample of individuals with Down's Syndrome of the proper age to reach clear-cut conclusions in any reasonable length of time. By pooling our resources and patients on a national basis, it is possible to dramatically shorten the time period for determining which medical or educational programs are of value in Down's Syndrome.

Improperly conducted medical or educational research treatment programs have two equally bad effects. First, parents are given false, optimistic expectations as to what the results will be for their child. It is only after many years of false anticipation and disappointment that the parents realize their expectations will not be reached. Secondly, a useful treatment program in Down's Syndrome could be totally missed if it were not conducted in such a way that a scientific evaluation of the program could be made.

REFERENCES

1. Bardon, L. M. E.: Siccacell treatment in mongolism. *Lancet* 2,234, 1964.
2. Benda, C. E.: *The Child With Mongolism.* New York: Grune and Stratton, 1960.
3. Berg, J. M., Kirman, B. H., Stern, J., and Mittwoch, U.: Treatment of mongolism with pituitary extract. *J. Ment. Sci.,* 107, 475, 1961.
4. Bumbalo, T. S., Morelewicz, H. V., and Berens, D. L.: Treatment of Down's Syndrome with the "U" series of drugs. *J. Amer. Med. Ass.,* 178, 361, 1964.
5. Collman, R. D., and Stoller, A.: A life table for mongols in Victoria, Australia. *J. Ment. Defic. Res.,* 7, 53, 1963.
6. Diamond, E. F., and Moon, M. S.: Neuromuscular development in mongoloid children. *Amer. J. Ment. Defic.,* 66, 218, 1961.
7. Hall, B.: Mongolism in newborns; a clinical and cytogenetic study. Lund: Berlingska Boktryckeriet, 1964.
8. Haubold, H., Loew, W. and Haefele-Niemann, R.: Possibilities and limitations of a post-maturation treatment of retarded and especially of mongoloid children. *Landarzt,* 36, 378-383, 1960.
9. Hunt, N.: *The World of Nigel Hunt.* Beaconsfield, England: Darwen Finlayson, Ltd., 1967.
10. Koch, R., Share, J., Webb, and Graliker, B. V.: The predictability of Gesell developmental scales in mongolism. *J. Pediat.,* 62, 93, 1963.
11. Koch, R., Share, J., and Graliker, B. V.: The effects of cytomel on young children with Down's Syndrome (mongolism): A double-blind longitudinal study. *J. Pediat,* 66:776, 1965.
12. Levinson, A., Friedman, A., and Stamps, F.: Variability of mongolism. *Pediatrics,* 16, 43, 1955.
13. Loeffler, F., and Smith, G. F.: Unpublished observations. 1964.
14. de Moragas, J.: Treatment of mongolism with dehydroepiandrosterone. *Rev. Esp. de Ped.,* 14, 493, 1958.
15. Oster, J.: *Mongolism.* Copenhagen: Danish Science Press Ltd., 1953.
16. Penrose, L. S.: The incidence of mongolism in the general population. *J. Ment. Sci.,* 95, 685, 1949.
17. Penrose, L. S., and Smith, G. F.: *Down's Anomaly.* London: J. & A. Churchill Ltd., 1966.
18. Stern, J. and Lewis, W. H. P.: The serum cholesterol level in children with mongolism and other mentally retarded children. *J. Ment. Defic. Res.,* 1, 96, 1957.
19. Turkel, H.: Medical treatment of mongolism. *Proc. 2nd Int. Cong. Ment. Retard.,* Vienna, 1, 409, 1963.
20. White, D., and Kaplitz, S. E.: Treatment of Down's Syndrome with a vitamin-mineral-hormonal preparation. *Int. Copenhagen Cong. Sci. Study Ment. Retard.,* 1, 224, 1964.

10

The Use of 5-Hydroxytryptophan in Patients with Down's Syndrome

MARY COLEMAN, M.D.

INTRODUCTION

Abnormalities in blood levels of serotonin have been reported in a number of types of mental retardation. It is very striking that there are a large number of disease entities associated with mental retardation where the blood level of serotonin in the patient is either abnormally high or low. An example of a disease entity with a low level of serotonin is phenylketonuria. An example of a disease entity with a high level of serotonin is hypothyroidism.

In these retardation syndromes the serotonin level in the blood moves from the abnormal range toward the normal range when these patients are placed on the proper treatment for the disease entity. For example, in phenylketonuria when the patients are placed on a low phenylalanine diet the serotonin level rises more toward the normal range (5). Conversely, when infant hypothyroid patients are given replacement thyroid therapy, the high serotonin level drops down into the normal range (2).

It was knowledge of these data that led us to our present attempt to normalize the blood serotonin levels in patients with Down's Syn-

The 5-HTP project discussed in this paper is the result of the joint efforts of many people, particularly Ann Barnet, M.D., Ann Lodge, Ph.D., and Leon Cytryn, M.D. Details of this study were published in the monograph, *Serotonin in Down's Syndrome*, North Holland Publishing Company, Amsterdam, 1973.

drome. First we studied the endogenous levels of serotonin in the blood of these children. We had the opportunity to study samples of 174 patients with the trisomy 21 form of Down's Syndrome, and a matching 174 normal children. We used the whole blood total 5-hydroxyindole (5-HI) method. In the normal newborn children, the mean 5-HI value under 24 hours of age was 73 nanograms/ml. Then the values declined 15% to a new low between 36 to 48 hours of age, and rose thereafter, achieving the childhood baseline level by 21 days of age. In the matched patients with trisomy 21, the mean 5-HI value under 24 hours of age was 34% lower than the value for the normal children of the same age. The values then rose more slowly than normal to a maximum level of 95 nanograms/ml. at two months of age. Instead of remaining at this baseline as in normal children, the 5-HI level in the Down's Syndrome children fell to another new low of 49 nanograms/ml. by five months of age. This low level is only 40% of the level of normal children. This level persists throughout childhood for trisomy 21 patients, and can slowly fall even lower as they grow older.

Thus, during the first two months of life, patients with trisomy 21 mimic the 5-HI pattern of normal children at a lower level and a slower pace. Between two and five months of age, the 5-HI value falls to a new, very low trisomy baseline which is maintained throughout childhood.

We also had an opportunity to study the 5-HI levels on 12 patients each, with the translocation and mosaic forms of Down's Syndrome. These levels were not significantly different from those of the trisomy 21 patients of the same ages. We studied two patients who had double chromosome errors; that is, they showed the presence of trisomy 21 and a second chromosome error. These two patients had 5-HI values higher and neurological examinations closer to normal than the trisomy 21 patients. Phenotypical mongols (that is, patients who clinically resemble other Down's Syndrome children, but who have completely normal chromosomes) have 5-HI values which are similar to those of normal children.

EFFECTS OF 5-HYDROXYTRYPTOPHAN VS PLACEBO IN DOWN'S SYNDROME

In conjunction with a number of other investigators, primarily Ann Barnet, M.D., Ann Lodge, Ph.D., and Leon Cytryn, M.D., we initiated an intensive, three-year double-blind study of the effect of 5-hydroxytryptophan treatment on Down's Syndrome. We had 19 patients in this study, starting in the newborn period. Half of the patients received the amino acid precursor to serotonin, 5-hydroxytryptophan, and the other half were given placebo. The study was done on a double-blind basis so that neither the parents nor the investigators were aware which children were receiving the amino acid.

The Mental Development Quotient (MDQ) of the Bayley Infant Scale for the patients receiving 5-hydroxytryptophan, and for those receiving placebo was not statistically different at one, two, or three years of age. This portion of the Bayley developmental scales appeared unaffected by the 5-hydroxytryptophan administration. Thus, there was no evidence that 5-hydroxytryptophan had any effect on intelligence, either positively or negatively.

The Psychomotor Development Quotient (PDQ) of the Bayley Infant Scale, which is primarily a measure of motor function, appeared to be affected by 5-HTP administration. At 12 and 14 months of age, the PDQ scores were significantly lower in patients receiving 5-hydroxytryptophan, showing a negative effect, although there was no statistically significant difference at 3 years of age.

The tonus scores, as determined by neurological examination, also showed a 5-hydroxytryptophan effect. An increase in tonus was noted in newborns receiving the amino acids, compared to placebo patients, for the first 3 months of life. After that age, tonus scores reversed and became lower in patients receiving 5-HTP for the rest of the study. Again, at 3 years of age the tonus scores in both 5-HTP and placebo patients were identical. These results suggest that 5-HTP does, in fact, affect systems mediating tonus, and that the effect may be positive at early ages and negative in later age groups.

The most interesting findings of the studies resulted from the analysis of the factors affecting tonus in Down's Syndrome, other than

5-HTP. It was very clear from the study that the "attitudinal effect" of the mother was a primary factor in affecting tonus. The tonus in young infants who were in adverse environmental situations, such as depressed or rejecting families, could not be improved with large doses of the amino acids without raising the doses to toxic levels. On the other hand, the tonus in young infants who were in very positive, accepting environments responded easily to 5-HTP and, in fact, could be improved merely by environmental factors.

One of the major conclusions of our study relates to the depression and despair that pediatricians induce in the parents of Down's Syndrome patients by informing them at birth of the coming disability of their child. A general rule for physicians states "if you cannot help, don't hurt." The whole area of informing and supporting parents regarding the diagnosis and prognosis of a Down's Syndrome child during the early months of life is identified by this study as an area which needs research.

In the initial 5-hydroxytryptophan studies in our clinic (1), we noted improved muscle tone which later led to what we assumed was an earlier age of walking (average age 22 months) than had been reported in the literature (3, 4). However, in the 5-HTP and placebo comparison study, the same early age of walking (22 months) was duplicated in the placebo patients. In fact, probably by coincidence, four out of nine of the placebo patients walked by 16 months of age.

Elaborate studies with the electroencephalogram, using background auditory potentials and visual evoked responses, were completed on the 5-HTP and placebo patients. One patient on the L-form of 5-HTP developed the infantile spasm syndrome and the EEG was hypsarrhythmic. Another patient who received the D, L-form of 5-HTP had hypsarrhythmic EEG, but no clinical seizures. The auditory and visual evoked potentials showed abnormal characteristics in both the placebo and 5-HTP patients. The auditory potentials particularly tend to be of higher amplitude in patients receiving 5-HTP. At the three-year evaluation, abnormal EEG's were significantly associated with lower Bayley PDQ scores, but not with MDQ scores.

Another very interesting finding in the study was the fact that the pretreatment serotonin levels correlated significantly with the six-month MDQ and PDQ scores, suggesting that the status of this biochemical measure may possibly be a predictor of early behavior development.

Introduction of the 5-HTP had no discernible effect on baseline temperature patterns in the neonatal period, the amount and severity of strabismus, the presence or severity of cardiac disease, or growth in height, weight or head size. We also could show no difference in the tongue protrusion or buccal-lingual abnormalities of this syndrome.

Biochemically, the most interesting finding of the study was the statistically significant elevation of epinephrine in the urine of the patients chronically receiving 5-HTP compared to placebo patients. Other catecholamine metabolites (norepinephrine, homovanillic acid, vanilmandelic acid and 3-methoxy-4-hydroxyphenylglycol) were not statistically different.

SUMMARY OF RESULTS OF 5-HYDROXYTRYPTOPHAN IN DOWN'S SYNDROME

From the information gathered, on the double-blind study of patients that received 5-HTP, compared with other patients in the clinic who received 5-HTP, a series of findings was available:

5-HTP does not improve the intelligence quotient in Down's Syndrome. A serious chronic effect of 5-HTP is the development of the infantile spasm syndrome which occurred in 14% of all patients who received the amino acid in the clinic. In most cases the syndrome was reversible by lowering or stopping the dosage of 5-HTP. ACTH treatment was required to reverse the EEG and clinical symptoms in one case. Acute side effects of 5-HTP are diarrhea, hyperactivity, opisthotonus, hyperacusis and hypertension. The acute side effects were reversible by lowering the dosage of 5-HTP. However, in ambulatory patients, too rapid a rate of withdrawal of 5-HTP is associated with ataxia.

In summary, our research with 5-hydroxytryptophan has led us to conclude that it is not indicated for use in treatment of Down's

Syndrome patients. At present we are studying other ways of raising serotonin in this patient group. A double-blind study comparing patients receiving Vitamin B_6, in large doses starting in the newborn period, to patients receiving placebo, is underway in our clinic at this time.

REFERENCES

1. BAZELON, M., PAINE, R. S., COWIE, V., HUNT, P., HOUCK, J. C., and MAHANAND, D.: Reversal of hypotonia in infants with Down's Syndrome by administration of 5-hydroxytryptophan. *Lancet*, 1, 1130, 1967.
2. COLEMAN, M.: Serotonin levels in infant hypothyroidism. *Lancet*, 2, 365, 1970.
3. DONAGHUE, E. C., KIRMAN, B. H., LABAN, D., and ABBAS, A.: Age of walking in the mentally retarded. *Int. Assoc. for the Scientific Study of Ment. Def. Proc.*, First Congress, Montpellier, France, 1967.
4. LEVINSON, A., FRIEDMAN, A., and STAMPS, F.: Variability of mongolism. *Pediatrics*, 16, 43, 1955.
5. MCKEAN, C. M.: Effects of totally synthetic, low phenylalanine diet on adolescent phenylketonuric patients. *Arch. Dis. Child.*, 46, 608, 1971.

11

The Use of 5-Hydroxytryptophan in the Treatment of Down's Syndrome

PHILLIP WEISE, PH.D., RICHARD KOCH, M.D.,
KENNETH N. F. SHAW, PH.D., *and*
MARTIN J. ROSENFELD, M.D.

INTRODUCTION

The treatment of children with Down's Syndrome with 5-hydroxytryptophan (5-HTP) was reported by Bazelon and colleagues (1) in 1967. Their report stimulated our interest in assessing the efficacy of this substance in our clinic. The rationale for its use is related to the fact that children with Down's Syndrome are said to have decreased blood levels of serotonin (5-hydroxytryptamine, 5-HT) (2, 3). Figure 1 outlines the metabolic pathway from 5-HTP via serotonin to 5-hydroxyindoleacetic acid (5-HIAA), the major excretory product in urine. It seemed reasonable to attempt elevation of serotonin levels to see what clinical effect this might produce. Since these children are nearly always mentally retarded, it was assumed that improvement in development would be the most sensitive indicator of clinical benefit. The purpose of this article is to report a study of 19 children with Down's Syndrome treated with 5-HTP from early infancy until three to four years of age.

Supported in part by the U. S. Department of Health, Education, and Welfare (grant No. MCHS-911, HD-1594 and RR-86), and a gift from the International Chemical and Nuclear Corporation.

FIGURE 1

TRYPTOPHAN (Trp)

↓ Tryptophan-5-hydroxylase — Argentaffin cells (intestine), brain, liver

5-HYDROXYTRYPTOPHAN (5-HTP)

↓ Aromatic L-amino acid decarboxylase — Kidney, adrenal, nerve tissue

5-HYDROXYTRYPTAMINE (5-HTA) (SEROTONIN)

↓ Monoamine oxidase — Liver, kidney

5-HYDROXYINDOLEACETALDEHYDE

↓ Aldehyde oxidase — Liver

5-HYDROXYINDOLEACETIC ACID (5-HIAA)

Main metabolic path for 5-hydroxyindole compounds.

METHODS

Twenty-six infants and children were initially selected at random for a clinical trial of 5-HTP. The clinical diagnosis of Down's Syndrome was verified by chromosome analysis, and trisomy 21 was confirmed in each patient. Six patients failed to complete the course of therapy, and one older child was excluded because her age (5 years) deviated considerably from the average age of the other patients (7 months). The final experimental group included 14 females and 5 males; 18 were Caucasian, and one was Oriental.

Pure 5-hydroxy-*DL*-tryptophan* was administered orally. Only the *L*-isomer is utilized biochemically, and the *D*-form is excreted in the urine unchanged for the greater part. The initial dose varied from 0.5 to 1.5 mg/kg/day and was increased as tolerated in a stepwise fashion using 1 mg/kg/day increments. The children were seen for medical evaluation at intervals of one to four months and were monitored regularly during home visits by a public health nurse. Developmental assessments utilizing the Gesell Developmental Schedules were performed at six to 12-month intervals. Urine samples were obtained at each visit for chromatographic determination of D-5HTP, 5-HIAA, tryptophan and other amino acids. In addition, urinary pH, volume and creatinine were measured. If urinary excretion of D-5HTP and 5-HIAA was non-detectable or showed no change from the previous sample, the dose was increased. Only if clinical symptoms of flushing, irritability or diarrhea occurred was the dose reduced.

RESULTS AND DISCUSSION

Clinical

5-HTP was well tolerated in the dose range used. Infantile spasms reported by Coleman (5) were not observed. Occasionally a subject had loose stools which ceased when the 5-HTP intake was decreased. No distinctive long-term improvement in muscle tone was noted in any of the patients over the course of treatment with 5-HTP.

---

* 5-hydroxy-DL-tryptophan was provided by the International Chemical and Nuclear Corporation.

FIGURE 2

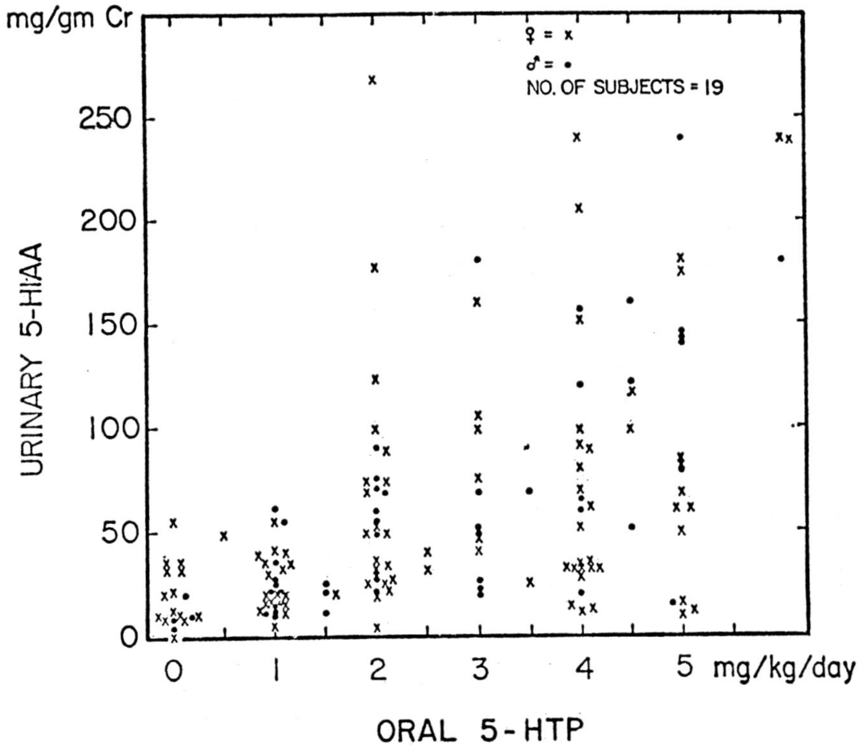

Urinary excretion of 5-hydroxyindoleacetic acid in relation to oral intake of 5-hydroxytryptophan in patients with Down's Syndrome.

The urinary excretion of 5-HIAA (shown in Figure 2) correlated well with the level of 5-HTP intake, as anticipated because 5-HIAA is the major urinary metabolite of 5-HTP.

Psychological

In this study each child's level of development was assessed through the use of Gesell Developmental Schedules which measure four major areas of behavior: Motor, Adaptive, Language and Personal-Social. The assessment was then recorded as a total Develop-

TABLE I

DQ's for Down's Children Treated With 5-Hydroxytryptophan

Case No.	*Age (months)*		*Development Quotient*		
Males	*Initial*	*At Completion*	*Initial*	*At Completion*	Δ
1	6	42	69	49	—20
2	24	35	62	56	— 6
3	4	44	65	43	—22
4	8	38	46	54	+ 8
5	3	52	77	52	—25
Females					
6	16	44	62	48	—14
7	8	50	59	39	—20
8	2	37	100	51	—49
9	5	48	40	43	+ 3
10	6	37	75	49	—26
11	7	51	70	49	—21
12	6	42	75	50	—25
13	2	33	67	55	—12
14	5	36	80	50	—30
15	7	34	70	49	—21
16	18	37	55	45	—10
17	2	45	57	42	—15
18	9	59	78	61	—17
19	9	51	86	51	—35

mental Quotient (DQ). The DQ's for the 19 children who completed the full course of 5-HTP treatment are shown in Table 1. The mean developmental quotients are reported for five age categories: Group I, ranged from 2-9 months; Group II, 14-24 months; Group III, 28-36 months; Group IV, 38-48 months; and Group V, 49-60 months (Table 2). These age categories conformed with those reported in an earlier study of the longitudinal development of Down's Syndrome infants and children (6). Our data were first analyzed by applying a t-test of the difference between these mean DQ's and the independently derived mean DQ's for each age category obtained by Share, et al. in their study of Down's children. The results of this analysis are found in Table 2. None of the differences was statistically significant for any of the five age categories.

Next our data were analyzed by comparing the initial and completion mean DQ's for our experimental group, in terms of sex

TABLE 2

Comparison of Gesell Mean DQ's of Experimental Group (5-HTP) with Independent Down's Group for Five Age Categories

Comparison Group	N	Mean DQ	SEm*	t	Sig.
Group I, 2-9 months					
Experimental	16	70	3.9	0.52	N.S.
Independent	45	68			
Group II, 14-24 months					
Experimental	10	58	2.7	0.00	N.S.
Independent	45	58			
Group III, 28-36 months					
Experimental	4	60	6.4	1.42	N.S.
Independent	45	51			
Group IV, 38-48 months					
Experimental	11	48	1.58	1.26	N.S.
Independent	45	46			
Group V, 49-60 months					
Experimental	5	52	2.50	0.67	N.S.
Independent	45	49			

*Standard error of the mean

TABLE 3

Comparison of Initial and Completion Gesell Developmental Quotients (DQ) of Experimental Group (5-HTP)

Comparisons	N	Initial DQ	Completion Mean DQ	MD	σMD*	t	Sig.
Males	5	64	51	13	6.18	2.10	N.S.
Females	14	70	49	21	3.30	6.32	Sig <.01
Males & Females	19	68	49	19	2.95	6.37	Sig <.01

*Standard Deviation of Mean Differences.

TABLE 4

Comparison of Experimental Group (5-HTP) With Independent Down's Group on Initial and Completion Gesell Developmental Quotients (DQ's)

Comparisons	N	Mean DQ	SD	SEm	t	Sig.
Initial DQ's						
Experimental						
Males	5	64	11			
					—0.77	N.S.
Females	14	70	15			
Experimental Males & Females	19	68				
				3.30	0.00	N.S.
Independent Group	45	68				
Completion DQ's						
Experimental						
Males	5	51	5			
					0.72	N.S.
Females	14	49	5			
Experimental Males & Females	19	49				
				1.18	2.55	Sig.
Independent Group	45	46				($p < .05$)

(Table 3) and also in comparison with the independent group of Down's children (Table 4). Comparison of the experimental group's initial and completion DQ's indicates a significant difference at the .01 level, with the mean difference being 19 DQ points lower after a mean 5-HTP treatment time of 35.2 months. A significant lowering of DQ in Down's infants with the passage of time has already been well documented (4, 6).

The results in Table 4 show that when the entire experimental group (N=19) is compared with the independent group (N=45) the completion mean DQ's are 3 points higher for the experimental group. This small improvement was statistically significant because of the small variability, or error in the mean DQ at the completion. It is important to note, however, that clinically this is indeed a very small improvement which results in no discernible behavioral differences suggestive of overall improved development. These results have been confirmed independently by Dr. Coleman and her co-workers (7) as well as by Partington, MacDonald and Tu (8).

CONCLUSION

In our opinion these findings indicate that the long-term systematic use of 5-HTP is not effective in increasing the overall rate of development of Down's Syndrome children as measured by the Gesell Developmental Schedules.

REFERENCES

1. BAZELON, M., PAINE, R. S., COWIE, V. A., HUNT, P., HOUCK, J. C., and MAHANAND, D.: Reversal of hypotonia in infants with Down's Syndrome by administration of 5-hydroxytryptophan. *Lancet,* 1:1131, 1967.
2. ROSNER, F., ONG, B. H., PAINE, R. S., and MAHANAND, D.: Blood-serotonin activity in trisomic and translocation. *Lancet,* 1:1191, 1965.
3. TU, J., and ZELLWEGER, H.: Blood-serotonin deficiency in Down's syndrome. *Lancet,* 2:715, 1965.
4. SHARE, J., KOCH, R., WEBB, A., and GRALIKER, B.: The longitudinal development of infants and young children with Down's Syndrome (mongolism). *Am. J. Mental Def.,* 68:685, 1964.
5. COLEMAN, M.: Infantile spasms associated with 5-hydroxytryptophan administration in patients with Down's Syndrome. *Neurology,* 21:911, 1971.
6. SHARE, J., WEBB, A., and KOCH, R.: A preliminary investigation of the early developmental status of mongoloid infants. *Am. J. Mental Def.* 66:238, 1961.
7. COLEMAN, M.: *Serotonin in Down's Syndrome.* Amsterdam: North Holland Publishing Company, 1973.
8. PARTINGTON, M. W., MACDONALD, M. R. A. and TU, J.: 5-hydroxytryptophan (5-HTP), in Down's Syndrome. *Develop. Med. Child Neurol.,* 13:362, 1971.

12

Decreased ATPase, Increased Na^+ and Decreased K^+ in Down's Syndrome Platelets

ERNEST E. MCCOY, M.D., DAVID J. SEGAL *and* KEN STRYNADKA

SUMMARY

Studies were undertaken to explain previous observations of decreased content and rate of uptake of serotonin into Down's Syndrome platelets. The inward transport of serotonin (5-HT) into rat platelets is coupled to the inward transport of Na^+. A decrease in platelet ATPase activity leads to an increase in Na^+ content which in turn results in decreased rate of Na^+ and serotonin uptake. In D.S. platelets a significant decrease in ATPase activity was observed as well as a significant increase in Na^+ and decrease in K^+ content. These data could account for decreased 5-HT content and uptake in Down's Syndrome platelets. The uptake of 5-HT in platelets has been proposed as a peripheral model for 5-HT uptake in brain synaptosomes; if decreased ATPase activity and increased Na^+ content occurred in D.S. synaptosomes, they might significantly affect neuronal transmission.

INTRODUCTION

Platelets from Down's Syndrome (D.S.) subjects have decreased serotonin content (1) and a decreased rate of serotonin (5-HT) uptake (2). Our previous studies (2) have shown that although ATP content is decreased in D.S. platelets, the ratio of the content of ATP/5-HT is increased in D.S. compared to normal. Synthesis of ATP from adenine is increased but that of ADP and AMP is similar in D.S. platelets (2). The results of these studies showed that the availability of ATP would not be a limiting factor in storage of 5-HT in D.S. platelets.

Studies by Sneddon on rat platelets have shown that the uptake of 5-HT is sodium-dependent (3); thus the inward transport of 5-HT is coupled to the inward movement of a sodium molecule. The continued inward movement of Na^+ in the platelet is coupled to the outward transport of Na^+, an energy-dependent process linked to the enzyme ATPase (4). Inhibition of this transport ATPase activity by ouabain results in an increase in intraplatelet Na^+ and a decreased inward transport of 5-HT (4).

This information on ATPase activity and Na^+ content was utilized in planning studies on Down's Syndrome platelets, to determine if the observed decreased rate of 5-HT uptake and content could be associated with decreased ATPase activity and increased Na^+ content in D.S. platelets.

METHODS

Platelets were isolated, the number determined by electronic particle counting, and then assayed for either ATPase activity or Na^+ and K^+ content. ATPase activity of platelet sonicates was determined by measuring ^{32}P cleaved from $AT^{32}P$ under optimal conditions of substrate level, time and amounts of Mg^{++}, Na^+ and K^+. The enzyme required Mg^{++}, was stimulated by K^+, and was inhibited approximately 50% by ouabain at 1×10^{-4}M concentration. Na^+ and K^+ contents of platelet pellets were determined by flame photometry, and corrected for plasma Na^+ and K^+ by the addition of ^{14}C-inulin to the platelet-rich plasma.

TABLE I

Sodium-Potassium Content of Platelets and Serum
D.S. and Normal Subjects

	μg $Na^+/10^9$ pl.	μg $K^+/10^9$ pl.	K^+/Na^+	mg Na^+/100 ml plasma	mg K^+/100 ml plasma
Down's Syndrome n=11	7.25±0.53	13.72±0.50	1.96±0.10	328.±5.1	21.09±1.59
Normal n=10	3.00±0.33	20.05±1.08	7.46±0.98	328.8±5.0	21.05±1.98
t	6.78	5.32	5.54	0.57	0.04
p	<0.001	<0.001	<0.001	>0.5	>0.5

RESULTS

1. *Sodium and Potassium Content of Platelets*

The average Na^+ content of platelets from 10 normal subjects was 3.00 μg/10^9 platelets, significantly different ($p<0.001$) from the average Na^+ content of platelets from 11 D.S. subjects of 7.25 μg/10^9 platelets (Table 1). The potassium content of normal platelets was 20.05 μg/10^9 platelets but that of D.S. platelets was reduced to 13.72 μg/10^9 platelets, also significant with $p<0.001$. The K^+/Na^+ ratio, or the amount of K^+ available relative to Na^+, was reduced in D.S. platelets; in normal platelets this ratio was 7.46 but in D.S. it was reduced to 1.96 ($p<0.001$). Thus there is a reduction in the amount of K^+ relative to Na^+ in D.S. platelets. There were no differences in total Na^+ plus K^+ content (i.e. total monovalent cation concentration) between D.S. and normal platelets, nor were plasma Na^+ and K^+ values different.

2. *Na^+ - K^+ - Activated, Mg^{++} - Dependent, Ouabain-Inhibited ATPase Activity of Platelets*

The average ATPase activity of platelet homogenate from 12 normal subjects was 181.0 nmoles cleaved/10^8 platelets/hour. In con-

TABLE 2

Platelet ATPase Activity: Normal and D.S. Subjects

	ATPase (nmoles AT32P cleaved/hr/108 platelets)
Down's Syndrome n=11	143.8±5.3
Normal n=12	181.0±6.6
t	4.38
p	<0.001

trast the average platelet ATPase activity from 11 D.S. subjects was 143.8 nmoles cleaved/10^8 platelets/hour. The lower ATPase activity of D.S. platelets was significant (Table 2) at $p<0.001$.

DISCUSSION

The uptake and storage of serotonin into platelets have many similarities to uptake and storage of serotonin into synaptosomes of the central nervous system (5), and the uptake and storage of 5-HT into platelets have been discussed as a peripheral model for these processes in brain synaptosomes (5, 6).

The results presented show that in D.S. platelets the Na^+ content is markedly increased, K^+ decreased and ATPase activity decreased. Sneddon has shown that the addition of ouabain, an ATPase inhibitor, to a suspension of rat platelets results in a decrease in ATPase activity, an increase in platelet Na^+ and a decrease in uptake of 5-HT. Conversely, when an increased inward transport of Na^+ occurred, there was also a marked increase in inward transport of 5-HT (4). To date, there has been no adequate explanation for the decreased serotonin content or rate of uptake in D.S. platelets. The present results may explain both decreased 5-HT uptake and 5-HT content of D.S. platelets, on the basis that decreased ATPase activity in D.S. platelets results in decreased outward transport of Na^+ and increased Na^+ content. The increase in platelet Na^+ content results in decreased inward movement of Na^+, and an accompanying decrease in the inward movement of 5-HT. As the rate of egress of

5-HT in D.S. platelets is normal, the net result is a decrease in 5-HT content. This sequence of reactions could account for both a decrease in V_{max} and content of serotonin described in D.S. platelets (1, 2).

If amine uptake into platelets is a model for amine uptake into brain synaptosomes, the following speculation is proposed: decreased ATPase activity may be present and increased Na^+ content occur in D.S. synaptosomes. This in turn would result in decreased amine content and decreased reuptake of amines after synaptic discharge; such a decrease in amine content and reuptake could possibly affect synaptic transmission and central nervous system function in D.S. patients.

REFERENCES

1. McCoy, E. E., Rostafinsky, J. J. and Fishburn, C.: The concentration of serotonin by platelets in Down's Syndrome. *J. Ment. Def. Res.* 12: 18, 1968.
2. Bayer, S. M. and McCoy, E. E.: Serotonin uptake and adenine nucleotide metabolism in platelets of Down's Syndrome patients. *Biochemical Medicine*, Vol. 9, 225, 1974.
3. Sneddon, J. M.: Sodium-dependent accumulation of 5-hydroxytryptamine by rat blood platelets. *Br. J. Pharmacol.* 37: 680, 1969.
4. Sneddon, J. M.: Relationship between internal Na^+/K^+ and accumulation of ^{14}C-5-hydroxytryptamine by rat platelets. *Br. J. Pharmacol.* 43: 834, 1971.
5. Paasonen, M. K.: Platelet 5-hydroxytryptamine as a model in pharmacology. *Ann Med. Exp. Fenn.* 46: 416, 1968.
6. Iverson, L. L.: Role of transmitter uptake mechanisms in synaptic neurotransmission. *Br. J. Pharmacol.* 41: 571, 1971.

13

Theoretical Concepts of Early Intervention

SIEGFRIED M. PUESCHEL, M.D., M.P.H.

After a lecture the late Francis Whalen Parker, a great Chicago educator, was questioned by a woman, "How early can I begin the education of my child?" The professor in reply asked, "When will your child be born?" "Born?" she said, astonished, "Why, he is already five years old." "My goodness," he shouted, "Don't stand there talking to me—hurry home, already you have lost the best five years" (1).

The underlying concern expressed in Francis Parker's message to this lady is also the central theme of this chapter, which will analyze some previous work in early development and explore certain aspects thereof, upon which new concepts of comprehensive care and stimulation of the young child with Down's Syndrome are based.

IMPACT OF ENVIRONMENTAL EXPERIENCES

Professionals experienced in the rapidly expanding field of human genetics are well aware of the lasting imprints of inherited factors on the developing organism. Of equal importance are aspects pertaining to the extent of the influence that environments may exert and the manner in which this influence may be expressed.

This investigation was supported in part by MCHS Project 928 and by NICHD Grant HD 5341-03, United States Department of Health, Education and Welfare.

In order to discern the impact of environmental experiences upon maturational processes, one should gain insight into evolving neurophysiological and psychological-social functions of the developing individual. In particular, the role of various sensory systems, including visual and auditory perception, imprints deriving from taste and smell, as well as tactile exploration and kinesthetic needs of the young child, should be studied as they relate to motor, mental, and language development.

During the past decades our understanding of these subjects has broadened considerably as a result of new information and research dealing with child development. Thus we have learned that during the first few years life moves at a rapid pace, never to be equaled in a like period. The young child's pattern undergoes a continuous transformation; he constantly is shedding habits or modifying them, and each child has a tempo and style of growth which are characteristic of his individuality.

In viewing the developmental progress of a normal child we must ask whether certain laws of sequence and maturation which account for general similarities and basic trends of child development also apply to the mentally handicapped, such as the child with Down's Syndrome. There are only a few absolutes to guide us, and we will have to look for the principles that are inherent in all development.

A study of the pertinent literature, including research with young animals, evaluations of natural experiments of deprivation, discerning observations and novel investigations of the development of the young child, reveals that one of the basic variables influencing later life is the quality and quantity of stimulation the young organism receives.

Animal Research

Well planned animal research has shown that the effect of experiences in early life is significant for later development and successful environmental adaptation in many species. Thus Levine (2) demonstrated that stimulation of infant rats accelerates the maturation of their central nervous system. The manipulated animals exhibited a more rapid rate of development and achieved motor coordination at an earlier age when compared with the nonstimulated animals.

Rosenzweig and co-workers (3) found that rats, kept in an enriched environment for 30 days, showed distinct changes in brain anatomy and chemistry, when compared with animals from a dull environment. The stimulated animals had greater weight and thickness of cortical tissue and an increase in total acetyl-cholinesterase activity of the cortex.

Shapiro and Vukovich (4) investigated the effects of a wide range of sensory stimulation on the development of cortical pyramidal cell synaptic loci in rats. They found an increase in the numbers of dendritic spines in stimulated animals.

Many similar studies in animals have yielded equivalent results. Inevitably, one has to raise the question whether the findings from animal experimentation are applicable to human beings. Although one must be careful in attempting to bridge the gap between animal studies and human biology, animal research raises questions and allows us to test concepts and theories, some of which may later prove useful in the research with human subjects.

Natural Experiments of Deprivation

Further evidence in support of the theory that experiences in early life have an important impact upon later development derives from "natural experiments of deprivation." Published reports point out that infants reared in psychologically inadequate institutions suffered serious defects in both the cognitive and emotional aspects of development.

Spitz (5) contrasted the development of infants living in a foundling home with children reared in a prison nursery. While the physical care was excellent in the foundling home, babies were kept in curtained cribs with no opportunity to establish warm contact with an adult human being. On the other hand, infants living in the prison nursery spent some time each day with their mothers receiving considerable affection and care. It was Spitz's conclusion that lack of love and stimulation was an adverse factor in institutional care which led to severe emotional disturbance and physical deterioration in those children.

The work by Bowlby (6) also emphasizes the importance of the presence of the mother in early childhood for satisfactory emotional adjustment. In another investigation of psychological privation in infancy and subsequent adjustment, Goldfarb (7) found that infant deprivation results in a basic defect of total personality. This defect manifests itself in the spheres of intellect and feeling in a manner suggesting that the institution child's personality is congealed at a level of extreme immaturity.

Of further interest is the report by Dennis (8), who compared the behavioral development of young children in three institutions. While in one of the institutions children were frequently handled and well cared for, children in the other two facilities were poorly attended. The motor development of children in the latter two institutions was significantly retarded when compared with the motor development of the subjects from the former residence.

Piaget's Concepts of Assimilation and Accommodation

Many developmental psychologists undoubtedly have been influenced by Piaget's keen observations of and investigations into the cognitive development of the young child (9). Piaget's theory is based on the concept of adaptation which is described as an interplay of two complementary processes: assimilation and accommodation. He calls the process of absorbing and organizing experiences around the activities that produce them assimilation, which is always being modified by an accompanying process which he terms accommodation. While assimilative processes constantly extend their domain, at the same time accommodation steers them toward ever more successful adaptation to the world. These dual processes, and the endeavor to maintain an equal balance between them, are the chief controlling factors of intellectual growth. According to Piaget the informative contact with the environment plays an important role in the development of prehension, and the expression of intelligent behavior in later life has its roots in the schemata laid down during the earliest months of life.

In keeping with Piaget's theory, it would be of importance during early age to provide an optimal environment for assimilation and to create situations which alter the activity patterns of the child, thus benefiting the process of accommodation.

Based on Piaget's work, enrichment studies were initiated by White and co-workers from the Harvard Laboratory of Human Development (10) which featured the special arrangement of physical circumstances and activities in which the infant lived. These enrichment procedures included extra handling, swiping at appropriate objects, visual exploration and prehension, and the provision of interesting and developmentally appropriate forms and objects in the infant's immediate surroundings. According to these studies, primary sensory-motor development, such as visual exploration, hand regard, and visually directed reaching, appears to be very sensitive to change in rearing situations. White demonstrated that major effects on the rate of development may be induced with ease by altering the infant's environment.

EARLY INTERVENTION PROGRAMS

Early intervention programs have been developed in many parts of the country during the past years (11). The rationale of the majority of these projects is based on the concept that environmental manipulation can alter the course of development in a young child and on the substantial evidence of the crucial importance of the early years in the maturation of personal competence. Most of these programs are dealing with normal or "disadvantaged" children; only a few reported studies initiated early stimulation of retarded children.

Bricker at the George Peabody College for Teachers recently started a research program which is structured to devise and evaluate various aspects of educational intervention in moderate to severe developmentally handicapped children (12). Rynders in Minnesota is engaged in a project assessing the effectiveness of tutoring on the development of the receptive and expressive language skills in young children with Down's Syndrome (13).

There are three other programs for young children with Down's Syndrome from abroad which should be mentioned briefly: Coriat (14) from Buenos Aires, Argentina offers "intensive stimulation" in the first year of life to a group of infants with Down's Syndrome. She found, using the Gesell method of assessment, that there is a significant difference between the IQ of the stimulated children and the IQ of the children in the control group.

Also, Ludlow (15) from Birchington, England is engaged in a study which investigates the effect of early intervention on the development of young children with Down's Syndrome. Children in her experimental group who received some stimulation were found to have an IQ consistently higher than those in the control group.

Brinkworth (16) from Birmingham, England compared a group of children with Down's Syndrome who were subjected to "maximal stimulation" during the first six months of life with a group of "unstimulated" children with the same disorder. His results showed a considerable advantage to the experimental group in social adjustment, motor performance, and mental abilities.

While the outcome of the latter three studies in scientific terms is unknown they demonstrate that theoretical considerations as discussed above can be translated into effective stimulation programs for children with Down's Syndrome.

SUMMARY

A basic understanding of developmental maturation and processes of deviation is the foundation upon which concepts of early educational programs can be developed. Although it is risky to extrapolate from a rat to a human, animal experiments have consistently demonstrated the importance of early stimulating experiences. When small children are deprived of maternal interaction and stimulation, intellectual and emotional dysfunction are observed. White's investigation and other studies found an enhanced developmental progress in infants placed in a stimulating environment. This would be of benefit to the innate assimilative process using Piaget's system. There are some promising programs for children with Down's Syndrome emphasizing the advantages of introducing environmental stimuli in early life.

REFERENCES

1. GESELL, A.: *The First Five Years of Life.* London: Methuen & Co., 1966.
2. LEVINE, S.: A further study of infantile handling and adult avoidance learning. *J. Personality,* 25: 70, 1956.
3. ROSENZWEIG, M. R., BENNETT, E. L. and DIAMOND, M. C.: Brain changes in response to experience. *Scientific American,* 226: 22, 1972.
4. SHAPIRO, S. and VUKOVICH, K. R.: Early experience effects on cortical dendrites: a proposed model for development. *Science,* 167: 292, 1970.
5. SPITZ, R. A.: Hospitalism: An inquiry into the genesis of psychiatric conditions in early childhood. In: *The Psychoanalytic Study of the Child,* Eissler, R. S. et. al. (Eds.), Vol. 1. New York: International Universities Press, 1945.
6. BOWLBY, J.: *Maternal Care and Mental Health.* Geneva: World Health Organization, 1952, Monograph Series No. 2.
7. GOLDFARB, W.: Psychological privation in infancy and subsequent adjustment. *Amer. J. Orthopsychiat.,* 15: 247, 1945.
8. DENNIS, W.: Causes of retardation among institutional children: I. *J. Genet. Psychol.,* 96: 47, 1960.
9. PIAGET, J.: *The Origin of Intelligence in Children.* New York: W. W. Norton, 1963.
10. WHITE, B. L.: *Experience and Psychological Development.* Englewood Cliffs, N. J.: Prentice-Hall, 1971.
11. BATTLE, C. U. and ACKERMAN, N. C.: *Early Identification and Intervention Programs for Infants with Developmental Delay and Their Families.* The Easter Seal Society for Crippled Children and Adults, Chicago, 1973.
12. BRICKER, W. A.: Personal communication, 1974.
13. RYNDERS, J.: Personal communication, 1974.
14. CORIAT, L. F.: Personal communication, 1974.
15. LUDLOW, J. R.: Personal communication, 1974.
16. BRINKWORTH, R.: Personal communication, 1974.

14

Principles and Methods of Early Intervention

ELIZABETH ZAUSMER, M.ED., P.T.

In the 1930's and 1940's much research centered on the effect of early experience on the child's development (1). During the following decade this interest decreased, to be revived in the late 60's when the Head Start Programs began. It became apparent that a child's experiences in early life—long before the Head Start age—are most crucial building stones for subsequent development in sensory-motor perception as well as in problem-solving. Many psychologists and educators (2, 3, 4, 5, 7, 8, 9) now believe in the importance of early experience. Experience may be regarded as programming the intrinsic portions of the cerebrum for present and future learning and problem-solving; in turn, learning may be conceived as the outcome of the nature and quality of the programming.

Normal development follows basically a direction which is hierarchically integrated and structured. It incorporates previous experience and matches already existing data with newly incoming information. It is an interaction of organism and environment. Structures develop through use and function, although the basis of such function is biologically determined. Thus, each stage in development is a precursor and preparation for another stage to come; acquisition of

This investigation was supported in part by MCHS Project 928 and by NICHD Grant HD 5341-03, United States Department of Health, Education and Welfare.

skill in one system brings about changes in the use of a different system.

While such developmental processes are now fairly well understood in infants and young children whose "normal" development follows a typical course, we know less well how they occur in children who are atypical and, in particular, who are mentally retarded.

One of the first questions we have to ask ourselves is whether developmental sequences are different in children with Down's Syndrome. It seems the answer is "no." In cases where the sequence of development is altered we should ask if this could be due to some additional defect, such as cardiac problems.

To a considerable extent the motor developmental delay is due to the hypotonia, particularly in the muscle groups needed to maintain anti-gravity positions. The child with Down's Syndrome frequently starts life with already inefficient or even distorted movement patterns: one finds weak sucking reflexes, insufficient head control with the resultant inability to lift or turn the head and to follow visual and auditory stimuli, and inadequate movements of the trunk and extremities resulting in faulty feedback of sensory experiences.

PLANNING AN EARLY STIMULATION PROGRAM FOR THE DOWN'S SYNDROME CHILD

An increase in sensory-motor input achieved through a specifically structured stimulation program provides additional and stronger stimuli. It elicits more definite responses and raises the level of attention. Hence, adequate sensory experiences motivate the child to repeat successful acts and to derive pleasure from them.

But the early sensory-motor program is only the starting point for a broad program of meaningful total stimulation. While the "normal" child does not need extensive instruction as he progresses toward more advanced and more complex intellectual goals, the child with lower physical and mental potentials seems to have a somewhat different pattern of learning. The child with Down's Syndrome is more apt to make a generalized response, to find it difficult to inhibit inappropriate responses and, particularly, to maintain adequate attention. Therefore, learning material must be broken down into smaller segments. Undesirable patterns of motor and other areas of behavior should be modified while the child is very young and the various systems are still plastic enough to allow for changes more readily than would be possible at a later stage of development.

But, while it is true that a child with Down's Syndrome learns better in a carefully structured situation and by imitation and frequent repetition, one has to guard against the tendency to offer only rote, stereotyped, repetitive, mechanistic learning experiences. Such models of instruction encourage automatic responses and result in ineffective cognitive patterns. For example, the parent who reports with pride that the child will sit for hours and play with the same toy, or likes to hear the same story over and over again, does not channel the child into more challenging learning experiences. Thus, it may well often be true that mentally retarded children do not learn to the full extent of their potential capacity because they are not sufficiently and effectively taught how to learn. We should be particularly aware of the basic and fundamental principles of learning —that changes in perceptual input are needed to attract attention— and that attention is a basic ingredient of learning. We can set the stage for effective changes in behavior, be they in the motor, cognitive or social developmental areas.

An assessment of the child's functional level—a careful analysis of the assets in the various areas of development and, primarily, as accurate an impression as possible of the child's global potential, as well as limitations—should precede the start of a program. Such assessment should be repeated at appropriate intervals to serve as basis for changes in the stimulation program. In our study the child is evaluated at birth and at age 3, 6, 9, 12, 18, 24 and 36 months. The parents are instructed how to carry out a stimulation program which is geared to the developmental level and the particular needs of the child (6).

When is the best time to start a stimulation program? The answer is the earlier the better. Frequently the child with Down's Syndrome does not receive attention and stimulation early enough. The infant who does not demand much time and attention is often mistakenly considered "good" by the parents. Often, parents interpret the hypotonia of their child as frailty. They might be afraid to handle the infant vigorously and, as a result, they deprive the child of much needed activity and stimulation. Unless there are pertinent medical reasons, the young child with Down's Syndrome should not only be exposed to the activities offered to the normal child, but should be given added opportunity to move, exercise, explore, play and learn—starting during the first few weeks of life.

We also must consider the timing of the various phases of an intervention program. The concept of the so-called "critical periods," as applied to overall development, has not yet been fully explored (10). Experienced professionals working with young children realize that there is a span of time in which the individual child responds best to, and derives most benefit from, a given learning situation. It is true that early experiences have multiple effects, but there is also ample evidence that there are periods of time during which an organism is particularly sensitive to specific developmental modifiers. It is at such periods that a specific part of an intervention program will prove to be most effective.

In addition to considering the level of readiness at which the individual child is best able to learn a given activity, it is important to give some thought to the methods of stimulation used at various stages of the child's physical, mental and social development. At one stage the child may derive greater benefit from demonstration or from strictly structured and supervised practice; at another stage, a less rigidly set situation may encourage learning by trial and error; and again, later, rational, deductive processes of learning should be encouraged. For example, the mentally retarded child presented for the first time with a formboard may profit merely by observing how the pieces are placed in the slots, or by touching the outlines of the pieces and the slots, or by being guided through various other sensory-motor experiences to place the pieces accurately. Later, only occasional directions or corrections may be needed to channel the child into more advanced learning, until, finally, he is able to make his own, internal comparisons and decisions and profits most from playing on his own. Thus, not only the content and level of the instruction, but the transmission, the timing, as well as the frequency of the learning experience, are changed according to the needs of the child.

AN EARLY STIMULATION PROGRAM

Following is a short presentation of concrete and practical aspects of our program. During the first few weeks of life, movements of the head are encouraged—first, through stimulation of rooting and sucking reflexes, followed by various changes in body positions which bring into play reflexive movements of the head and trunk and necessitate the use of anti-gravity musculature. The prone lying position is suggested at rest time; during the waking hours the infant is frequently held suspended horizontally and vertically and is tilted into a variety of directions. Such activities elicit labyrinthine and proprioceptive equilibrium reactions and responses and bring into play muscle groups which otherwise are apt to remain inactive if the child is always held in supported positions.

During the first few months we use tactile stimuli, such as touching, stroking, and tapping, to elicit more active movements of the head, trunk, and the extremities. Guided assisted movements are combined with visual, tactile and auditory stimuli. The infant soon learns to associate such movements with sensory, pleasant experiences and he is apt to choose them as a model for more active, spontaneous participation.

Unfortunately, the child with Down's Syndrome is often left for long periods in the crib or in the playpen where, at best, he can roll over to get at his toys; he might be placed in a high chair with a back support, or sit on the floor with the legs widely abducted, outwardly rotated, the back excessively rounded and head hanging forward. These positions are detrimental to the acquisition of more "normal" motor development, leading to good patterns of sitting, creeping and standing. Furthermore, they prevent the child from making use of his full potentials to look around in all directions, to handle an object at an appropriate distance for visual-tactile exploration, preparing for more advanced motor and cognitive learning experiences. We suggest, for instance, that even the very young child be sat on a low chair, his feet resting on the floor. In this position, the back most often will be held up straight. A small table or box placed in front makes it possible to keep the arms at an optimal level for play. This also provides a better angle for visual exploration and encourages some shifting of the weight onto the legs.

In the context of this brief description of our program more detailed methods and techniques used to provide adequate experiences in subsequent stages of gross and fine motor development cannot be presented. It should be mentioned that the parents are fully instructed not only in the "how to do" aspects of the program, but also in regard to "why" a particular approach is followed. They are also given written instructions. Parents are advised about appropriate play material, and how to use it most effectively. It is suggested that they devote a period of time regularly and specifically to a training session and that they keep a record of progress.

The parents are the most important factor in the stimulation program. Without the full cooperation of the family, any remedial program is doomed to failure. On the other hand, parents who become positively and actively involved in the care and training of their child are able to cope more adequately with their own feelings and they are better able to accept their child's limitations. Parents who, through this kind of work, engage in frequent physical contact with their child provide not only much needed stimulation, but also emotional support. The child, in turn, reinforces their positive attitude by responding in tangible ways, such as smiling, vocalizing, embracing and, more generally, accepting their wishes and directions. In such an atmosphere of give-and-take, emotional and behavioral problems seldom arise; if they do, they most frequently can be remedied.

RESULTS OF STIMULATION PROGRAM

We cannot yet come to any definite, statistically supported conclusions with regard to the effectiveness of the stimulation program which began 3 years ago. Yet, we have observed that with stimulation and training, started as early in infancy as possible, one can influence the trend of sensory-motor, social and most likely, also, cognitive development in children with Down's Syndrome. As was to be expected, we have found a wide range in the level of function, even at the first examination of the newborn and, particularly, in the rate of improvement and in the degree of competency and cooperation of the family. Only more time and the analysis of extended data will give us exact answers to the many specific questions related to the rate of acquisition of developmental milestones through a stimulation program.

At this point, we can only report that we are pleased and encouraged with the achievement of our group of children. We already see that many of the abnormal motor characteristics frequently found in the child with Down's Syndrome can be avoided. We find that motivation and initiative to engage in more challenging activities can be increased and that the groundwork for a more efficient learning "set" can be laid out early. Thus, undesirable behavioral traits can be avoided or remedied in infancy and early childhood. It is apparent that parents derive a great deal of support from the program and that the children have a happy start in life.

We hope also to be able to demonstrate that the old stereotyped view that most children with Down's Syndrome have severe limitations and are unable to learn is quite unjustified and, as a matter of fact, untenable.

REFERENCES

1. ULICH, R.: *History of Educational Thought.* Boston: American Book Co., 1945.
2. CALDWELL, B.: The rationale for early intervention. *Exceptional Children,* 36: 717, 1970.
3. HUNT, J. McV.: *Intelligence and Experience.* New York: Ronald Press, 1961.
4. CALDWELL, B. M. and RICHMOND, J.: The Children's Center in Syracuse. In: L. L. Dittman, Ed., *Early Child Care: The New Perspectives.* New York: Atherton Press, 1968.
5. BUTLER, A. L.: *Current Research in Early Childhood Education: A Compilation and Analysis for Program Planners.* Amer. Assoc. of Elementary-Kindergarten-Nursery Educators, 1970.

6. ZAUSMER, E., PUESCHEL, S. M. and SHEA, A.: A sensory-motor stimulation program for the young child with Down's Syndrome. *MCH Exchange*, 2: 1, 1972.
7. The President's Committee on Mental Retardation: Screening and assessment of young children at developmental risks. DHEW Publication No. (OS) 73-91, Washington, 1973.
8. GORDON, I. and LALLY, J.: *Intellectual Stimulation of Infants and Toddlers.* Gainesville: Univ. of Florida Press, 1967.
9. MEIER, J. H.: A survey of infant stimulation and intervention programs. In: *Parent Counseling and Infant Stimulation—Workshop Proceeding*, April 1972. Denver, Col.: Mountain-Plains Regional Center, 1972.
10. CONNELLY, K.: Learning and the concept of critical periods in infancy. *Develop. Med. Child. Neur.*, 14: 705, 1972.

15

Infant Stimulation

KATHRYN E. BARNARD, R.N., PH.D.

I would like to address the topic of programs for infant stimulation by posing three major questions. They are: What sparked the interest in working with young infants? What is the rationale for infant stimulation? And last, what questions and hence criteria should be applied to the evaluation of infant stimulation programs?

INITIATION OF INTEREST IN WORKING WITH INFANTS

Considering the first question of what initiated the interest in working with young infants, five events account for our current emphasis on early intervention. These are:

1. Success in teaching mentally retarded children. This success has largely come about through the application of behavioral modification theory and techniques which have helped us to specify with more precision goals, behaviors and processes by which the environment can be modified to help the individual attain progress.
2. Societal emphasis on family care and the development of support systems in the community to help families care for handicapped children in their own home.

During this study the investigator was supported by a Research Fellowship from the Division of Nursing, National Institutes of Health, United States Public Health Service, Department of Health, Education and Welfare. Dr. Helen Bee Douglas was the major faculty advisor during this fellowship. Research reported here was supported by a grant from the United Cerebral Palsy Research Foundation, 1971-72.

3. The Head Start movement and subsequent evaluation of intervention with preschool children from deprived environments which suggested that emphasis should be put on starting at earlier ages.
4. The increased knowledge of child development and its related fields as they pertain to the period of infancy.
5. Demonstration and research of many programs in the past ten years dealing not only with environmentally but also organically impaired children.

RATIONALE FOR INFANCY PROGRAMMING

From the generation of interest, we move to the important question of what the rationale is for programming during infancy. Studies dealing with the effects of deprived environments on the school performance of children suggest that the amount and type of stimulation the child experiences during his early years of life are important (8, 9, 10, 20). Investigations of persons such as Hess and Shipman (9); Bee, VanEgeren, Streissguth, Nyman, and Leckie (3); Yarrow, Rubenstein and Pederson (21); Porter (13); and Barnard (1) have also given us insight into what elements in particular seem to be important in the environments of children, and hence associated with later achievement. From the work of Hess and Shipman (9) and Bee et al. (3) we learned that the verbal interaction and language style of the mother were related to good or poor achievement of the child; specifically the mother who verbalized more and used abstractions in her verbalizations usually had a child with more verbal skill. In addition, the effect of maternal feedback was noted as important, in that the child who received positive contingent feedback on his or her learning attempts did better, while children who did less well had mothers who gave more negative reinforcement and less total positive reinforcement (3, 18).

Another study which begins to give a more in-depth explanation of the importance of stimulation during infancy is the work of Yarrow, et al. (21). In a study of five-month-old infants and their mothers, they evaluated the naturalistic environment (home) from the standpoint of the degree and type of inanimate and animate stimulation available to the child, and correlated this information with the infant's performance on the Bayley Scales of Infant Development. These findings represent one of the most detail measures of the infant's real world. They support the ideas that animate stimulation, mother or caretaker interaction, is linked to language development at this age, and the amount of inanimate stimulation is related to such cognitive skills as problem-solving behaviors in the infant. The measure of inanimate objects included everything in the child's proximal area. In addition to counting the objects, they coded them as to their complexity and the reactivity of the object to the infant's actions. The sheer variety of objects and their reactivity to the infant seemed to be the two important qualities of the infant's experience. It is logical that these qualities are important, particularly if you think of intelligence as the processing of information. The infant learns to handle more information, based on his previous experience with a variety of information processing episodes, such as inanimate objects. So much the better if they react to his actions.

Porter (13) reports an experimental study in which she had mothers provide passive exercise to their infants in the form of cycling movements of the arms and legs. Thus far, she has studied children in a United States foundling home and another group from the Philippines. The results, as measured by the Gesell Infant Scale, show significant gains for both groups, particularly in motor and language development. The gains in language development were marked and can perhaps be explained by the probable increase in animate stimulation that occurred as the result of the caretaker or mother doing the exercising. Porter's study should be examined because it represents the presentation of a simple technique which sets the stage for sensory-motor experiences for the young child and leaves the mother or caretaker free to initiate their own cultural pattern of interaction.

In testing out modalities of stimulation in premature infants, several investigators (1, 12, 14, 16), have shown that kinesthetic, tactile, and auditory stimulation has had beneficial effects on the growth and development of premature infants while still in the hospital incubator. Thus research with the youngest possible subjects, premature infants, shows that systematic attempts to facilitate the infant's growth and development by altering the environment do improve the infant's development. One particular study involved a program of rocking and heartbeat sounds for 15 minutes every hour (1). In addition to improving their sleep pattern and increasing early weight gain, follow-up data from infants in the study suggest that infants on the early program of rocking and heartbeat stimulation during their 34-35th week of gestational age had better growth over a year later (2).

Hence we get some notion of the tremendous indirect effect that early stimulation has on later behavior, in that it changes the behavior of the child early in infancy. This changed behavior—in the case of the study of premature infants, sleeping better and being more alert when awake—allowed them to be ready for interaction with their mothers and caretakers, thus setting off a whole cycle of increased interaction with people in their environment.

Another type of study, looking at which variables of pregnancy and early postnatal life are associated with later developmental or neurological difficulties (15), suggests the scores on the Bayley Scales of Infant Development, especially the scores at eight months of age on the motor component of the scale, correlate well with measures of cognitive skills at seven years of age. This is interesting to note since during this same time period, six to ten months of age, there is a rather large decline in test performance of Down's Syndrome infants, as documented by the studies of their mental and motor development (5, 7).

These three studies (5, 7, 15) concerning the predictiveness of motor development at eight months, and the rapid decline in performance of the Down's Syndrome infants, suggest that the early months are important and sensitive periods of the infant and young child's life. The normal child in an average environment probably does not require any additional programming since innate curiosity will provide an abundance of experiences. There is evidence to support the fact that infants who are in altered environments or infants who have some intrinsic biological alteration do benefit from a systematic approach and special attention to their environment during these early months (1, 2, 5, 6, 8, 10, 11, 12, 13, 17).

The modality of stimulation is not the important issue. It is more significant that the infant be in an environment which he can interact in and with. Gordon (8) has pioneered work with the whole question of early intervention, particularly working with both infants and parents. His work involves a very specific program of weekly visits into the home and instructing the parents in how to play games with the infant. The data indicate that the best results were obtained when the program was initiated and carried out in the first three years of life. However, it was interesting to note the children who did the next best were the group where the program was initiated and carried out during the child's first year of life. One possible explanation for this phenomenon is that the rapid changes that go on naturally during the first year of life put infant programming with the mother at a considerable advantage. As the mother did things with her child and noted changes, she was reinforced for her efforts and thus continued interaction with the child in the subsequent years, even without direction.

One must also ask whether the first year's enhancement of sensory-motor development is important in developing a child who is alert and ready for more interaction in the ensuing years. Bronfenbrenner (4) reported that early childhood intervention programs with the best outcome effects were those in which the emphasis of intervention was not only with the infant, but equally with the parent. In such programs the effects are not only lasting, but cumulative. Levenstein (10) developed a particularly interesting schema of having home visitors, whom she referred to as toy demonstrators, present toys to the mothers and demonstrate to them how to use the toy to play with the child. The idea of using the toy was to provide a situation and vehicle of promoting verbal stimulation and parent-child interaction. The results of her studies over a three- to five-year period indicate a 15 point test score differential in favor of the toy demonstration group, in contrast to a control group without the toy demonstration.

To cite examples of programs more closely related to the topic of this conference, that of Down's Syndrome infants, children and adults, I am familiar with two programs at the University of

Washington (19). One program involves an interdisciplinary team including a nurse, nutritionist, physical therapist, and pediatrician, working with Down's Syndrome infants and their parents. The approach has been to start with the parents' questions, concerns and interests about the child's development. From that point the parents are encouraged to expand their efforts with the child by group discussion and support from the team and other parents, and with demonstration of specific management or stimulation techniques. For instance, a mother may talk about the infant beginning to notice noises. The staff takes this occasion to encourage the mother to make sure that when the child does localize a sound he is taken to the sound and then introduced to other kinds of sounds as well, thus capitalizing on the child's interest. The results of this program are encouraging, and more detailed analysis has been done by Dr. Beverly VanderVeer, University of Washington, Child Development and Mental Retardation Center (19). To report the findings briefly, they have data with matched age subjects which demonstrate a significant difference between children in the intervention program, especially in the group with intervention prior to 30 months of age.

Similarly, at the Experimental Education Unit, another program of the University's Child Development Center, there is a program directed by Dr. Alice Hayden for Down's Syndrome infants and preschoolers. This program offers intervention guidance to keep the child's developmental progress in line with established developmental norms, such as the Denver Developmental Screening Test and the Gesell Infant Scales. Their results, coupled with the results of Dicks-Mireaux (7) and Carr (5), give good documentation that specific programs of stimulation are important for the biologically impaired child. Many people and groups are providing early intervention and stimulation for Down's Syndrome infants, all of which involve components of what has been outlined by Zausmer, Pueschel, and Shea (22). Their basic categories and illustrations are as follows:

Visual Stimulation:

> Provision of interesting and developmentally appropriate objects—differing in color, shape, and distance.

Optimal positioning to enable the child to make the best use of the visual equipment—particularly in the upright position.
Provision of experience in visual tracking as well as permanency.
Combining visual with other sensory-motor experiences.

Auditory Stimulation:

Introduction of sounds of variable quality, frequency and intensity—derived from different directions and distances.

Sounds reinforced with visual and tactile stimuli—particularly with facial expressions and gestures.
Repetition of sounds which the infant produces.

Additional Sensory Stimulation Relating to Sound Production and Speech:

Oral stimulation to encourage sucking, licking.
Oral stimulation to encourage closure of the mouth.
Oral stimulation to encourage tongue movements.
Oral stimulation to encourage chewing.

Kinesthetic Stimulation:

Frequent changes in body positions—particularly those which elicit vestibular reactions.

Activities which encourage symmetrical and alternate or reciprocal movement patterns appropriate to specific developmental stages.

To summarize, rationale has been provided for the importance of animate and inanimate stimulation for the infant, and in Down's Syndrome infants a drop in test scores between six and ten months of age, unequaled by losses at future time points, has been reported. Furthermore, evidence from VanderVeer's data (19) suggests that infants with Down's Syndrome, in a parent-child focused intervention program prior to 30 months of age, show the most favorable developmental progress. Data presented indicate that for the biologically and environmentally impaired child it is appropriate to advocate infant programming.

GUIDELINES FOR INFANT PROGRAMS

The issue of guidelines for infant programs is important since many people and agencies are involved, and more are becoming involved in early infant stimulation programs. The period of infancy is especially susceptible to change and likewise parents who have recently learned of their child's problem are in a sensitive reaction stage. Thus, programs should be planned with due regard to the powerful potential to influence behavior and later outcomes. The primary goal of any program should be to increase the satisfaction the parents and children derive from one another. A few questions are presented as examples of the issues from which guidelines or evaluation criteria could emerge:

1. *How are parents involved in the program?*

The research evidence indicates if we expect to see lasting and cumulative outcome effects on the development of the child, the parents must be active participants in the program, either in individual one-to-one sessions with the professional staff, or, perhaps even more effective, in parent group sessions where they can learn from and support one another.

2. *What systematic observation has been done with the child and family?*

It is essential that baseline data, or entry behavior of the infant as well as the parents and siblings, be sought. For the infant this would include information related to past and present attainment on scales of infant development, physical growth, and daily patterns of sleep activity. The parents should be interviewed by the staff to find out where they are in dealing with the situation and in general how they feel it is affecting them and their family. It is important to incorporate the parents' goals for the infant and the family into the programming at the initial contact with them by involving them in planning whatever programming is appropriate to the situation. Depending on the age of the siblings, information about their reactions and involvement should be obtained. Generally for the younger children this would come from the parents, and for school-age and older children, an interview with them would be appropriate. Often siblings are very involved in interacting with the infant.

As important as developmental information, attitudes and feelings of the parents and siblings is the observation of interaction between the persons involved: mother-infant; father-infant; sibling-infant; mother-sibling, and so forth. While it is probably not possible or necessary to collect samples of all family dyadic interaction, it is essential to have some observational data about interactions between the infant and the person who will be most involved in carrying out the specific stimulation. What feedback does the mother give the baby for attempting to reach for an object? How well does the baby attend when the parent is showing him how to put the spoon in the bowl? Does he make it worth her time to teach him? In situations where there is a negative feedback system operating, the first order of business is to help the mother or caretaker and infant to have positive and satisfying interactions.

3. *What individual programs are planned for the child and family?*

It has already been alluded to, but it is important to repeat, that one of the important programming aspects should focus on the parent-infant interaction. A mutually satisfying relationship will be the base for all other endeavors and is the key element in insuring that the programming stays operational even after the parents and infant are no longer associated with a specific infant stimulation program or agency. A "turned-on" parent will turn on the child and at this point the mutual feedback will maintain a good environment for the infant.

The second major area is sensory-motor stimulation. The outline previously cited by Zausmer provides a good summary of the general concepts. A note of concern should be voiced about over-stimulation. Many times we become overzealous in our efforts to increase the child's skills and attempt too much bombardment of stimuli or programming. The usual indication that this is happening is when the child becomes irritable and fussy. An important concept to keep in mind is the basic rest-activity cycle; we do best when we have alternate periods of activity and rest, or people and privacy.

4. *What parameters are used to evaluate the effectiveness of the program?*

In an effort to help the infant and change his or her behavior, evaluation efforts in the past have been heavily child-oriented. We need to develop and use more measures of the impact that early intervention has on parents and other family members. What happens to family unity, mobility, occupational changes, and the general mental health of the parents and siblings?

5. *What professional staff are involved and what supervision is provided for other mid-level staff?*

One effective concept is that one person can integrate the knowledge and skills of many disciplines and provide in a single staff member the primary contact for an infant and his family. This may mean that the teacher is providing not only the usual stimulation content, but also incorporating ideas of physical handling that will encourage the baby to use his muscles. Likewise, the psychologist may be giving the mother advice about the baby's diet as she directs the mother in a more positive feedback system with her infant. Evidence from Head Start programs has established the value of using trained paraprofessional staff in implementing the program. This fosters the extension of the professionals' knowledge and creates a mid-level staff person whose specific training related to the infant program can be well utilized by the parents.

6. *Where is the program based?*

Particularly for the child under 18 months of age, the programming effort should have as its ultimate focus the home situation. This is in contrast to the preschool model which considers the period in school as a primary element. In working with infants the staff seeks methods which will help the parent incorporate ideas into daily practices in the child's own home. The staff may go directly to the home, or the parents and infants may come to a center for the sessions. After 18 months the children often benefit from group interaction such as the normal preschool offers. Parents of any age child will profit from contacts with other parents. Many programs have parent groups as a regular element of their offerings.

7. *Can the staff support their activities with rationale?*

People involved with infants, children and parents should be aware of the importance of their actions on the child's and the parent's life and should be able to elucidate the theoretical underpinnings of their approach. This holds true for a program based in a university setting, as well as one based in the upper story of a small town Grange Hall.

Working with infants has become a popular activity, and well it should, for there is no better way to reduce the problems of a child with developmental deviancy than to provide the optimal climate for the habilitation of the developmental and personal interactional skills that will put the growing child in touch with the opportunities that exist in the world outside of the child's home.

REFERENCES

1. Barnard, K. E.: The effect of stimulation on duration and amount of sleep and wakefulness in the premature infant. Unpublished doctoral dissertation, University of Washington, Seattle, 1972.
2. Barnard, K. E.: A program of stimulation for infants born prematurely. Paper given at the Society for Research in Child Development, Philadelphia, March, 1973.
3. Bee, H. L., VanEgeren, L. F., Streissguth, A. P., Nyman, B. A., and Leckie, M. S.: Social class differences in maternal teaching strategies and speech patterns. *Developmental Psychology* 1: 726-734, 1969.
4. Bronfenbrenner, U.: Remarks made in presentation at the American Academy of Pediatrics, Chicago, 1973.
5. Carr, J.: Mental and motor development in young mongol children. *Journal of Mental Deficiency Research* 14(3): 205-220, September, 1970.
6. Centerwall, S. A. and Centerwall, W. R.: A study of children with mongolism reared in home compared to those reared away from the home. *Pediatrics* 25: 678-685, April, 1960.
7. Dicks-Mireaux, M. J.: Mental development of infants with Down's Syndrome. *American Journal of Mental Deficiency* 77(1):26-32, July, 1972.
8. Gordon, I. J.: The Florida Parent Education Early Intervention Projects: A Longitudinal Look. Research Reports, Institute for Develop-

ment of Human Resources, College of Education, University of Florida, Gainesville, 1973.

9. HESS, R. D. and SHIPMAN, V. C.: Early experience and the socialization of cognitive modes in children. *Child Development* 36: 869-886, December, 1965.

10. LEVENSTEIN, P.: Cognitive growth in preschoolers through verbal interaction with mothers. *American Journal of Orthopsychiatry* 40: 426-432, April, 1970.

11. MOORE, R. S. and MOORE, D.: How early should they go to school? *Childhood Education* 14-20, October, 1973.

12. NEAL, M. V.: Relationship between vestibular stimulation and the developmental behavior of the premature infant. Unpublished doctoral disertation, New York University, 1967.

13. PORTER, L. S.: The impact of physical-physiological activity on infants' growth and development. *Nursing Research* 21(3): 210-219, May-June, 1972.

14. SEGALL, M. E.: Cardiac responsivity to auditory stimulation in premature infants. *Nursing Research* 21(1): 15-19, January-February, 1972.

15. SMITH, A. C., FLICK, G. L., FERRISS, G. S., and SELLMAN, A. H.: Prediction of developmental outcome at seven years from prenatal, perinatal, and postnatal events. *Child Development* 43: 495-507, June, 1972.

16. SOLKHOFF, N., YAFFE, S., WEINTRAUB, D. and BLASE, B.: Effects of handling on the subsequent developments of premature infants. *Developmental Psychology* 1: 765-768, 1969.

17. STEDMAN, D. J. and EICHORN, D. H.: A comparison of growth and development of institutionalized and home reared mongoloids during infancy and early childhood. *American Journal of Mental Deficiency,* 69: 391-401, November, 1964.

18. STREISSGUTH, A. P. and BEE, H. L.: Mother-child interactions and cognitive development in children. In W. W. Hartup (Ed.) *The Young Child. Review of Research.* Vol. 2. Washington D.C. National Association for Education of Young Children, 1972.

19. VANDER VEER, B. and SCHWEID, E.: Infant assessment: stability of mental functioning in young retarded children. *American Journal of Mental Deficiency,* 79:1-4, 1974.

20. WERNER, E., SEMONIAN, K., BIERMAN, J., and FRENCH, F. E.: Cumulative effect of perinatal complication and deprived environment on physical, intellectual and social development of preschool children. *Pediatrics* 39(4): 490-505, April, 1967.

21. YARROW, L., RUBENSTEIN, J. L. and PEDERSON, F. A.: Dimensions of Early Stimulation: Differential Effects on Infant Development. *Merrill-Palmer Quarterly* 18:205-218, 1972.

22. ZAUSMER E., PUESCHEL S., and SHEA A.: A sensory-motor stimulation program for the young child with Down's Syndrome. Preliminary Report 2(4): December 1972. MCH Exchange, Department of Health Care Administration, The George Washington University, Washington D.C.

16

Language Intervention – Changing the Language Environment of the Retarded Child

SUE SEITZ, PH.D.

The language intervention program reported here is based on a view of mental retardation as one aspect of slow development, in which development follows a normal sequence, but at a rate which is delayed in comparison to the norm.

This position underlies some language intervention programs, notably that of Miller and Yoder (17), who argue that the content of language training for retarded children should be taken from the data available on language development in normal children, and that this content should be taught in the same sequence as it is acquired by the normal child.

This notion that children will acquire language best if the content is presented in the natural developmental sequence is extended here to propose that language also be presented as nearly as possible in the same context and by the same processes which support language acquisition in the child developing at a normal rate.

Theoretical orientations have important consequences for the design of intervention programs. The theorist who holds a defect position hypothesizes that the retarded child is different, rather than merely delayed, and that the child's difference or defect renders him incapable of profiting from the natural environment. Thus, it becomes necessary to create an artificial environment in which the child can learn.

A clinician working from a developmental position might argue that the environment most likely to prove effective and motivating for retarded children is composed of those ingredients which foster language acquisition in the normal child. These ingredients may not be available to the retarded child, however, unless the environmental response is tuned to the child's developmental level.

This raises some specific questions for a developmental treatment program:

1. What is the normal process and context of language acquisition?
2. Does the language environment of the child with delayed language differ from that of the normal child?
3. If so, can we change the language environment of the retarded child to the type of environment which supports language in his normal mental age peer?
4. And finally, if we could bring about such a change, would it have positive consequences for the acquisition and use of language by the child?

LANGUAGE ENVIRONMENT OF THE NORMAL CHILD

Let us begin by examining some of the available data on the language environment of the normal child. Ordinarily children acquire language in the course of interaction with their mothers. They learn to use vocalization first as signals, then as symbols, for contacting and communicating with this singularly significant person.

The way in which language is used for communication can be described best by the social and linguistic behaviors of the child and his mother. If we consider this interaction from the aspect of the social process we find that it is characterized by a high degree of reciprocity—that it constitutes a relationship in which each member of the dyad is a potent stimulus for the other.

Lewis and Freedle, in their 1972 monograph, *The Mother-Infant Dyad: The Cradle of Meaning* (15), conclude that, "The interaction of the infant and its mother reflects . . . a finely tuned and potentially meaningful system wherein each allows the other to act." They maintain that from birth there exists a communication network between the infant and his mother, and that language evolves from this network. They point to the manner in which this dyad maintains communication through vocalization, touch, and smile, linking these behaviors into communication chains which are steadily lengthened during the first year of life. They have documented some of the parameters to which infant vocalization is sensitive: female infants tend to vocalize more when their mother addresses her utterances to them, whereas male infants do not make such discrimination. Infants at 12 weeks vocalize differently in different environments: they vocalize most in the playpen and on the floor, least in the crib and lap. This may be partially attributable to being closer to mother in the latter situations, with mother talking more and the infant remaining quiet.

Moss (19) and Kagan and Lewis (10) have reported that mothers' voices have the effect of inhibiting speech in three-month-old infants, with more infant vocalizations occurring when mother is absent. This finding, however, is subject to socioeconomic status (SES) differences and holds only for middle SES (MSES) mothers. Children of lower SES (LSES) mothers vocalize more when mother is present and talking. In general, however, of all the parent-child behaviors, vocalization most often elicits vocalization from both mother and child.

Lewis and Freedle (15) followed three of their young subjects through age two and found that the children maintained the same rank order for vocal behavior they had held at 3 months of age, which suggests that some aspects of communicative behavior emerge very early and remain quite stable.

The ontogenesis of communicative behavior may in fact begin with the neonate. Thoman and her colleagues (27) report relationships between mother's response to crying and neonate's time to soothe, with soothing achieved most quickly when mother's response was under 90 seconds and when there was little variance in the mother's time to respond. Bell and Ainsworth (1) present some data from a longitudinal study of year-old infants which indicate that the infant learns from his mother's responses to crying that this behavior has communicative value. The learning does not seem to follow a simple stimulus-response pattern, however. When mothers respond to crying by holding the baby, the result is not to increase crying, but instead to decrease it. Babies of responsive mothers cried less and used significantly more noncrying forms of vocal communication at one year than babies of nonresponsive mothers.

Some socioeconomic differences are apparent in the pattern of mother-child interactions at ten months. LSES mothers vocalize to infants less than MSES mothers (28), although such maternal behavior would elicit more vocalizations from the LSES child if the early pattern detected by Lewis and Freedle persists. LSES mothers, however, believed their children were not capable of understanding, and therefore felt it was pointless to talk with them. This finding is only one of several recent publications pointing to the effect which the parent's perception of the child has on parental behavior (9, 21, 22).

The maternal social behavior most interwoven with the early development of communication between mother and child when the child begins to function independently is that of obtaining obedience or compliance. In a study of 9- to 12-month-old infants observed since birth, Stayton, Hogan and Ainsworth (25) found that the maternal behavior most predictive of infant obedience at this age was maternal sensitivity to infants' signals. The mother who responded to her child's efforts at communicating his needs was most likely to have a child who responded to her requests.

Terdal and Seitz (26) have reported a similar negative relationship between the amount of commanding by the mother and the degree of responsiveness by the child. Stayton et al. (25) define maternal qualities related to compliance as: sensitivity to the infant's needs; acceptance of him and his behavior; and cooperativeness, as opposed to interfering, in that the mother does not try to impose her will on the baby, but arranges her schedule to minimize interference with him. The interfering mother "assumes that she has a perfect right to do with (the baby) what she wishes, imposing her will on his, shaping him to her standards, and interrupting him arbitrarily without regard for his moods, wishes or activity-in-progress."

All three of these maternal qualities (sensitivity, cooperativeness, and acceptance) were highly and positively related to the infant's obedience to maternal commands. Thus, the responsive mother has a responsive infant. This has implications for social behaviors other than compliance, since communication, by its very nature, implies social responsiveness.

This relationship continues to hold for the two-year-old, according to Minton, Kagan and Levine (18). They report similar relationships between parental socialization methods and child obedience. While LSES mothers used more commands and prohibitions, their children were less obedient than children of MSES mothers. Moreover, the children of MSES mothers more frequently requested that their mothers play with them.

Olim (20) directly links mothers' controlling behavior to language and communication development:

> The consequences for the child of the mother's use of inhibitory and input-control techniques are to promote the development of a nonrational, nonverbal stance toward the environment. By cutting off the opportunity for the child to engage in linguistic and symbolic interaction, the results for the child are a limited repertoire of information and ideas . . . a low level of differentiation and complexity in his linguistic and cognitive structure (p. 222).

Therefore, in the relationship between a social, communicative two-year-old and his mother there is a general responsiveness to one another; the mother is attentive to the child, and the child actively engages the mother in his activities and generally complies with her requests.

What correlates of this social pattern can be found in the language behaviors of the normal mother-child (M-C) pair?

Broen (3) describes the environment of the language learning child in a study comparing the way in which mothers talked to their young (Mean CA=21 mos.) and older (Mean CA=60 mos.) children:

> In general, the mother's speech was slow, with pauses located always and only at sentence boundaries, when they talked with their younger children. They used a small vocabulary and often repeated what they had said, with and without variation. Mothers' sentences seemed to fall into two major sentence patterns. One pattern is built on the imperative sentence and . . . expands that form in a variety of ways. The other sentence pattern includes variations and permutations of a "be" sentence. Mothers also used single word and grammatically incomplete responses (p. 63).

Similar findings reported by Frank and Seegmiller (7) are based on a longitudinal study of children from two and a half to five years of age. They summarize their data by saying (p. 7):

> Mothers regularize and simplify their speech to their children. They monitor their speech less as their children get older and approach full mastery of the language. Mothers seemed unaware that they modified their language in accordance with their children's developmental level.

Snow's (24) article on mothers' speech to children learning language reports similar data for mothers addressing young (two-year-old) children, but an experimental manipulation allows additional insight into mother's linguistic behavior. Snow had mothers present instructions to their two-year-olds under two conditions: 1) when the child was absent, via tape recording; and 2) when the child was present. The presence of the child produced an immediate modification of maternal speech to accommodate comprehension. Thus, it would seem that mothers continuously monitor their children for signals of comprehension and modify their speech accordingly. These modifications produced for the young child "a sample of speech which is simpler, more redundant, and less confusing than normal adult speech" (p. 565).

Thus, looking at both social and linguistic aspects of the normal mother-child relationship, we find a dynamic responsiveness, with the maternal social and linguistic behavior matched to the child's needs and developmental level. The child, in turn, seeks the parent's companionship, and is generally compliant to her commands.

LANGUAGE ENVIRONMENT OF THE RETARDED CHILD

Let us turn now to an examination of data available on the interactions between a mother and her retarded child.

First, a note of caution. There is a paucity of normative data on this population, since most material is gathered in the course of clinical identification of mental retardation. It may be that there are families in which the mother is sensitive, accepting, and cooperative and is linguistically appropriate with her retarded child. The studies in this area, however, are unlikely to contain data from such families.

While there are considerable data on the language of retarded children, most of these data have been drawn from children in institutions and gathered by researchers who were relative strangers to the children—hardly the significant objects of communication that the mother would represent. Still, accumulating research shows that the language of the retarded child follows the same developmental sequence as the normal child, but at a slower rate (13, 14).

There are, however, few data, comparable to those on normals, from retarded children and their mothers on early vocalizations and communications.

Whitehurst, Novak and Zorn (29) employed the mother as the therapist for a retarded child. Working with a single subject in the home setting, they increased the child's rate of acquisition of new words significantly over 45 sessions. The authors point out that the purpose of the study was not to develop a therapeutic program, but to study language as a social process. The greatest rate of increase in new words was under a condition in which the parent used both prompts (naming objects) and a high level of conversation, a change from the mother's usual repertoire of few prompts and little conversation.

Marshall, Hegrenes and Goldstein (16) observed parents of retarded children and parents of normal children interacting with their youngsters in a free play situation. They report that the mothers of retarded children gave significantly more commands, asked more questions and used fewer intraverbal behaviors—that is, ordinary conversation and comments—than the mothers of the normal children. The authors ask, if these interactions were changed, would the verbal behavior of the retarded children change also? This paper offers some evidence that this is so. And yet, at the same time, the author disagrees with Marshall et al.'s interpretation of the mechanism supporting the mothers' commanding behavior. Marshall et al. argue that parental commanding behavior is maintained because it is reinforced by the child. This interpretation seems unlikely in view of the evidence that children whose parents overstructure and command are usually less compliant (11, 12, 18, 25). On the other hand, it could be argued that it is the mother's perception of her child that influences her response on several dimensions, social as well as linguistic. Osofsky and O'Connell's (21) research on perceived dependency is in accord with this, showing that when parents perceive a daughter to be more helpless in a task situation, they give more directions and assistance.

Terdal and Seitz (26) observed the same behaviors which Marshall reports, and demonstrated experimental shifts in M-C interactions through providing mothers with an opportunity to observe and imitate therapists interacting with their children in a play group setting. This approach, in which mothers practiced modeling the therapists' behavior, was more effective than an operant program designed to have the mother consequate a specific target behavior. (Part of the effectiveness of the modeling approach over the operant approach lay in its generalization to other than the target behavior. Parents who participated in the modeling program were more responsive to the child's play, and engaged in more interactions with their children. The children were less negative and more compliant).

AN EXPERIMENTAL PROGRAM

The data to be discussed today are collected to document what, if any, effect such changes in M-C interactions have on the language behavior of young, retarded children, and, secondly, to add to our knowledge of the language environment of the retarded child, with particular attention to ways in which it may differ from that of his normally developing language-age peer.

TABLE I

Children's Chronological Age, Developmental Age, Pre-Program and Post-Program Mean Length of Utterance

	C.A. (Post-test—months)	D.A. (Post-test—months)	MLU PRE	MLU POST
Group I				
S1	20.5	23	1.07	1.05
S2	24	24	2.01	1.94
S3	23	23	1.05	1.33
Group II				
S4	27	24	1.04	1.44
S5	41	24	1.50	1.82
S6	37	36	1.00	2.31

Method

Ss: Children in this study were obtained through two types of resources. Those children in Group II, the language delayed group, were referred from various clinics in the Madison area. The presenting problem was language delay, although in the case of two of the children formal testing was not possible because of behavior problems. The three *Ss* in this group were each in a different session of the treatment program and were drawn from a sample of eight language-delayed children who had participated in the program. The selection of these particular *Ss* for this report was constrained by the availability of an appropriate comparison group, the three *Ss* in Group I. Mothers of Group I children had requested that their children be allowed to participate so that they (the mothers) could observe the youngsters in group activities, as they were considering nursery school placement. The mothers were notified of the program through a community newsletter.

Children were matched on the basis of level of functioning in language as measured in the free play situation, using mean length of utterance (MLU) as a criterion. Other measures were not possible since the children in Group II were not testable at the time of entry. Scores on the Denver Developmental Screening Test (8) were obtained on all children following the program, and for S_6, in Group II, a score on the Peabody Picture Vocabulary Test, Form B (6), was also obtained since his language functioning still lagged other areas by six months. Post-test CAs for Group I *Ss* were 20.5, 24, 23 mos; Group II *Ss* were 27, 41, and 37 months (Table I).

Also shown in Table 1 are the *Ss* MLU for the pre- and post-tests. Pre-test measures show a MLU range from 1.00—2.01 words, with the extreme high score belonging to a 22-month-old girl in Group 1.

Two sets of parents in Group 1 and one set in Group II had attended college and worked as professionals or semiprofessionals. The other parents had no more than high school education and the fathers were employed in skilled or unskilled labor.

Procedure

All M-C pairs were videotaped for 15 minutes prior to and upon completion of the program. The parents and children were filmed in an unfamiliar room, in which there was a collection of age-appropriate toys. Instructions to mothers were: "I'd like you to play with your child as you would if you had a few minutes to spend with him or her at home." Immediately following both the initial and final filming sessions each parent was shown the video film, with the purpose of assessing parents' understanding and interpretation of their child's behavior. This method of sharing these video films helped establish a communication between parent and the investigator based on jointly observed behaviors.

Children and their parents came to the program for one hour a day three consecutive days per week for eight weeks. During the first six sessions, parents observed through the one-way mirrors as graduate students "played" with their children.

The student therapists had been trained to comment on the children's activities, to reflect and expand their utterances, and to engage them when possible in conversation and join in their play.

The only behavioral restriction placed on the children was the prohibition of physical aggression against self or others, for which the child had to spend time out in the hall.

Students were positively reinforced in the presence of parents for appropriate interactions with the children. Parents were reinforced by *E* and students for describing and engaging in positive behaviors of their children.

After the sixth session parents were given the option of going into the playroom, providing the children would consent, and providing they felt they could interact with the children in a manner similar to that of the student therapists. By the time the parents entered the playroom the children had begun to be self-initiating in selecting activities. During the last three weeks, parents substituted entirely for the student therapists.

Videotapes of the pre- and post-sessions were transcribed by two or more observers. When an utterance was not fully understood by all observers, it was scored as an Unintelligible Vocalization (UNV). (Definition of the utterance is that used by Snow (24).)

Transcripts were divided into 15-second intervals for purposes of time-sampling selected social and linguistic aspects of behavior.

RESULTS AND DISCUSSION

1. *Analysis of social behaviors*: The analysis of the social behavior was scored on a matrix (Figure 1). Children's behaviors are classified by the four categories on the Y axis; parental behaviors are listed on the X axis. A decision is made for each 15-second time frame as to the behavior of parent and child that characterized the interval: Thus, parent directs, child responds positively would result in a score in cell 15. Behaviors were conceptualized as co-occurring with no attempt made to specify the antecedent or consequent behavior for any behavior. No Response for the child, or Unrelated Response for the parent is scored only if no other behavior occurs.

Unrelated behavior on the part of the mother may be interpreted as behavior not involving the child's immediate activity, but which is designed to engage the child in some activity of the mother's by making it appear attractive, rather than by directing the child to participate. This category also reflects some instances when the mother was not in evidence on the videotape.

Measured on this matrix, the pre-test scores for Group I mothers showed an 80 percent compliance rate while Group II mothers had

		CHILD BEHAVIORS		
PARENT BEHAVIORS	NO RES	— RES	+ RES	INDEP PLAY
+ RES	1	2	3	4
— RES	5	6	7	8
UNRELATED	9	10	11	12
DIRECT.	13	14	15	16

FIGURE 1

a 43 percent compliance rate. Post-test scores show both Groups obtaining a 98% or better compliance rate, a significant difference from the pre-test, ($t = -2.677$, $df = 4$, $p < .05$). (One Group I mother was discarded from the analysis of compliance data since she gave no directives to the child and thus had a zero compliance score.)

Scores in the cell which reflects a positive response from both mother and child discriminated between the two groups of dyads on the pre-test (Mann-Whitney $U = 0$, $p = .05$), with Group I pairs

FIGURE 2

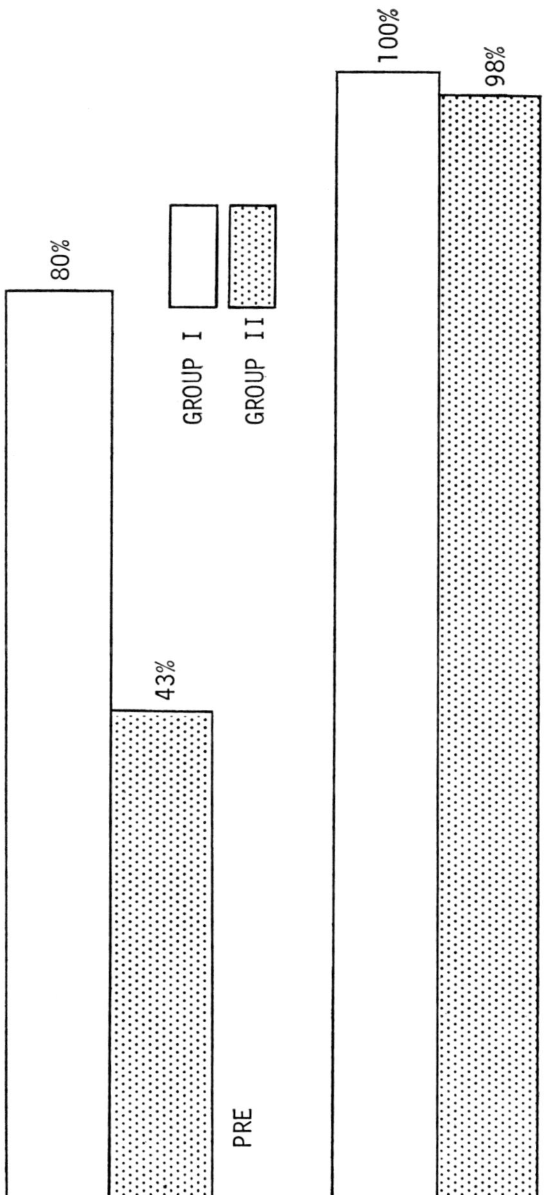

Child Compliance to Mother's Commands

TABLE 2

Children's Mean Number of Utterances, Pre-Post

	Group I	Group II
Pre	81.66	42.66
Post	117.	126.

having significantly more scores in this cell. Post-test scores showed a slight improvement in this behavior for the Group II mothers (pre-test M = 16; post-test M = 28.33, Mann-Whitney U = 2; p=.20). Group II mothers also increased the number of positive responses to the child's independent play, from 29% to 73%, the level at which Group I mothers functioned on entry to the program.

In summarizing the data on social behaviors, post-test scores show mothers and children responding more positively to one another when this is measured in behavioral terms.

2. *Analysis of linguistic behaviors*: Total utterances for both the mothers and children were counted. One mother in Group II had only one utterance on the pre-test. However, the scores of the other two mothers in this group (M=184) did not differ significantly from those of the mothers in Group I (M=191).

The number of total utterances for the two groups of children was sufficiently different so as to regard them as separate groups for pre-post comparisons (Mann-Whitney U = 2, p = .20; (23)). The Group II children showed a significant increase in total number of utterances on the post-test (Mann-Whitney U = 0; p = .05). There was no significant difference in the pre-post test scores for Group I *Ss* (see Table 2).

The concept that sharing time in a conversation is an index of how responsive participants are to one another is not particularly new. It was thus postulated that a conversation ratio of one-to-one would reflect a situation of maximum responsiveness, minimum control of the conversation. A conversation ratio was computed for each M-C pair, and the distance from 1:1 ratio was determined. This measure did not discriminate the two groups on the pre-test (Group I M ratio = 1.75; Group II M ratio = 1.78). However, both groups

TABLE 3

Percent* of Mother's Statements used as Commands, Comments, and Questions

	Group I		Group II	
	Commands			
	%	Ratio	%	Ratio
Pre	.14	80/573	.14	81/369
Post	.05	22/490	.06	18/331
	Comments			
Pre	.25	133/573	.18	98/369
Post	.40	196/490	.41	134/331
	Questions			
Pre	.23	135/573	.24	86/369
Post	.26	130/490	.21	71/331

*Percents are based on the mean of the summed individual percentages, not on the summed raw score ratio.

of M-C pairs significantly shifted their conversation ratio on the post-test towards the 1:1 ratio ($t = 2.10$, $df = 5$, $p < .05$.). Post-test means were 1.04 for Group I and .44 for Group II.

Moreover, the MLU of Group II children showed a significant increase over their pre-test scores (Table 1) with a pre-test mean of 1.18 and a post-test mean of 1.86 (Mann-Whitney $u = 1$, $p = .10$).

Children in Group I did not show a significant change in MLU, which is not surprising, since this measure is tied to developmental level. Neither the developmental level nor the language environment of these children was changed by the program. For the Group II children, however, some aspects of the language environment changed, permitting them to show an increment in performance more representative of their developmental level.

Four of the children increased their maximum length of utterance on the post-test, accounting for a significant increase in this measure for all child *Ss* ($t = 1.879$, $df = 5$, $p = .10$).

Thus, on the post-test, children were sharing conversation more equally and Group II children were producing somewhat longer utterances.

Utterances of the two groups of mothers were analyzed according to the proportion of utterances that were used as commands, comments and questions.

Commands are defined as statement-form utterances requiring a behavior from the child. (Question-commands were not included in this count.) Comments were defined as statements on the child's or mother's activity, and might include repetitions or expansions of the child's utterances. Tag questions were included in the comment category, e.g., "You have the dolly, don't you?" All other questions were counted separately.

Inspection of the data showed no differences between the two groups' mean ratios of comments, commands, or questions on the pre-test. Mothers were therefore treated as one group when analyzing post-test data on these particular measures.

Post-test means reflect a significant reduction in the ratio of commands used ($t = 1.64$, $df = 5$, $p < .10$) and an increase in the ratio of comments ($t = 4.54$, $df = 5$, $p < .005$), as shown in Figure 3. There was no difference in the ratio of questions used.

A further analysis was made of the number of times a mother's comment included a word or complete utterance of the child. The child's utterance had to occur in the speech immediately preceding the mother's. This analysis differs from Cazden's (5) in which the child's utterance would precede the mother's by three utterances. A repetition, or imitation, of the child's speech was scored as such if the word the child used was repeated exactly or included in a comment of the mother's. The latter was considered to be an expansion. Different forms of the word were not scored. Words repeated in the context of a question were not scored. The count of repetitions of the child's speech by mothers may therefore be somewhat lower than that provided by other researchers (e.g., Cazden (5), Brown and Bellugi (2)).

The mean number of repetitions of the two groups of mothers was judged sufficiently different on the pre-test to treat them as two different groups, although the probability level was only .20 (Mann-Whitney $U = 2$). On the post-test, the Group I mothers showed no significant change, but the Group II mothers had significantly in-

FIGURE 3

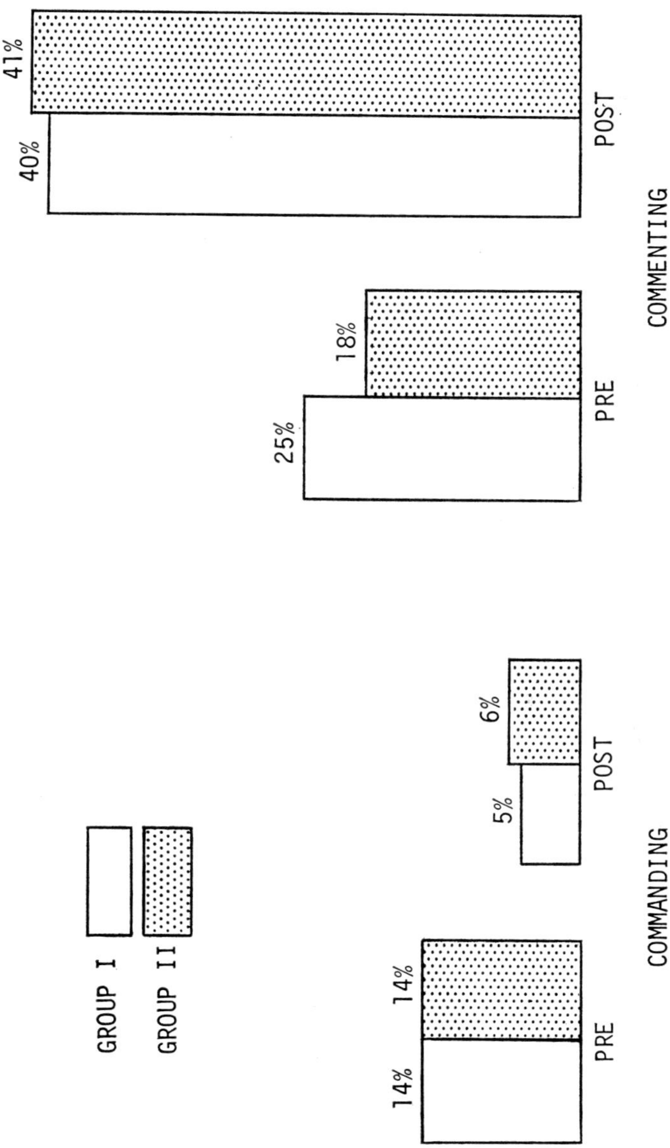

Percent of Mother's Total Utterances

TABLE 4

	Group I		Group II	
	% Child's Utterances Repeated by Mother			
	M%	Ratio	M%	Ratio
Pre	.24	63/251	.11	15/128
Post	.28	83/235	.18	33/253
	% Mother's Utterances Repeated by Child			
	M%	Ratio	M%	Ratio
Pre	.08	36/551	.02	16/369
Post	.09	44/468	.17	45/331

creased their repetitions of their children's utterances ($t = 7.18$, $df = 2$, $p < .01$).

A similar analysis was then made of the number of times children repeated mothers' utterances, as shown in Table 4.

Children in Group I maintained about their pre-test ratio of repetitions on the post-test, and the ratio of M-C repetitions for this group remained about 3 to 1. (Similar data on two normal M-C pairs has also been reported by Brown and Bellugi, 2).

For the children in Group II, however, there was a significant increase in the number of their mothers' utterance that they repeated (Mann-Whitney $U = 0$; $p = .05$) and the ratio of repetitions between the mother and child equalized, as shown in Figure 4.

Thus, one aspect of language behavior clearly discriminated between the two groups of mothers on the pre-test—the number of times they repeated or expanded on their children's utterances.

For both groups, however, and on both the pre-and post-tests, mothers repeat the child's utterances more often than children repeat the mother's utterances.

Cazden (5), in categorizing functions of adult responses to child speech, includes confirmation, which may simply be a repetition of the child's utterance. It is enticing to examine the role such confirmation could play in language acquisition.

Jerome Bruner, in his paper on "Competence in Infants" (4), details the growth of the infant's skill in grasping from the first athetoid arm motions to the mature, certain grasp. Bruner observes that there are distinct stages in the development of this skill and that

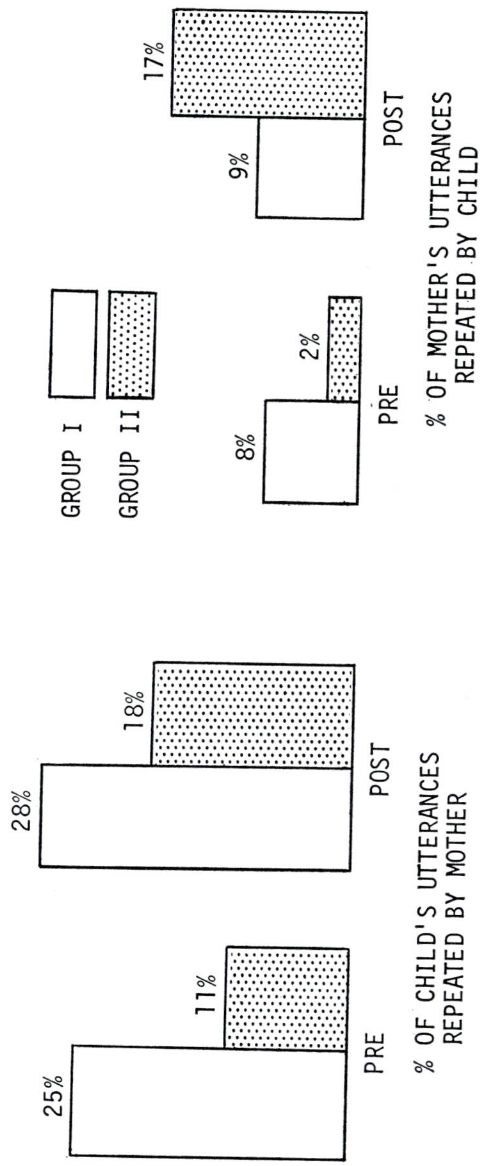
GROUP I
GROUP II
25%
11%
28%
18%
PRE
POST
% OF CHILD'S UTTERANCES
REPEATED BY MOTHER
8%
2%
9%
17%
PRE
POST
% OF MOTHER'S UTTERANCES
REPEATED BY CHILD

FIGURE 4

infants practice each stage until a pattern is mastered. They then abruptly discard the perfected pattern and proceed to build a new, amplified, more precise pattern using components of the old pattern, but varying their sequence or adding new components. It is as if the infant stores the perfected pattern in order to practice a new one, which may serve him less well at first, but which he will continue to practice until it also is mastered.

It may be that the mother's repetition of her child's word provides the feedback necessary to confirm a stage of mastery of that word, just as attainment of the desired object confirms that the intended grasping pattern was executed and was correct. The mother's repetition of the child's utterance could convey confirmation of one or all of several aspects of that utterance, such as:

a) correctness of the auditory signal;
b) correctness of its perceptual and cognitive referent;
c) an understanding of its communication intent.

The child then has confirmation of mastery of the word at some level, and can move to practice new patterns of this behavior, new words, and new combinations of words. This would explain the increase found in child's repetitions of mother's utterances which accompanies an increase in the mother's repetitions of child utterances. A series of parametric studies is being designed to further explore this notion.

It is further possible that the process of repeating the child's utterance also places a governor on the mother's MLU, which has been observed to increase with the increasing linguistic competence of the child. If this were found to be true, it would serve as one mechanism underlying the movement of the child from one stage of language to another. The child could be seen as incorporating new language forms and functions as he receives confirmation of his mastery of old ones, his own linguistic level always serving as a control on the linguistic input he receives from his mother.

Furthermore, it is not only confirmation of the auditory signal and its perceptual and cognitive referents that is important in this feedback, but also the communication intent. As Whitehurst et al. (29) point out (p. 175):

> Speech therapists, when discussing deprivation of stimulation as a cause of delayed speech, have tended to assume that deprivation has to be quite dramatic. The forest and orphanage are often cited as environments in which deprivation of speech input is likely to be important. Yet it is obvious that environmental deprivation can be a very subtle variable and yet have quite profound effects.

The data presented here seem to support their conclusion that verbal interaction is more crucial than verbal stimulation.

What are the implications, then, for language therapy for retarded children? First of all, since parental perceptions of the child may affect their interaction with him, one implication is that the parents may need to be trained to observe the child's behavior, and the functions it serves, and to react to that behavior and its functions and not to their perception of defect. This may be especially true where children are stigmatized and a stereotype is attached.

But this carries with it the implicit assumption that language therapy will involve that salient and significant aspect of the child's environment: the verbal interactions he has with his parents. Parents can be trained to use these interactions to respond positively to the child at his level of functioning so that they confirm his achievements and support new attempts at mastery.

REFERENCES

1. BELL, S., and AINSWORTH, M. D. S.: Infant crying and maternal responsiveness: Reinforcement reassessed. Unpublished manuscript, 1971. Cited in Lewis, M. and Freedle, R. *Mother-Infant Dyad: The Cradle of Meaning*. Princeton, N. J.: Educational Testing Service, 1972.
2. BROWN, R. and BELLUGI, U.: Three processes in the child's acquisition of syntax. *Harvard Educational Review*, 1964, *34*, 133-151.
3. BROEN, PATRICIA ANN.: The verbal environment of the language-learning child, *ASHA Monographs*, No. 17, 1972.
4. BRUNER, JEROME S.: Competence in infants. Paper presented to Society for Research in Child Development, Minneapolis, Minnesota, March, 1971.

5. Cazden, C. B.: Environmental assistance to the child's acquisition of grammar. Unpublished doctoral dissertation, Harvard University, 1965.

6. Dunn, Lloyd: *Peabody Picture Vocabulary Test.* Circle Pines, Minn.: American Guidance Service, Inc., 1959.

7. Frank, Sheldon M., and Seegmiller, M. S.: Children's language environment in free play situation. Paper presented to Society for Research in Child Development, Philadelphia, March, 1973.

8. Frankenburg, W. K., and Dodd, J. B.: The Denver Developmental Screening Test. *Journal of Pediatrics,* 1967, *71* (2), 181-191.

9. Kagan, J.: On class differences and early development. In Denenberg, V. H. (ed.) *Education of the Infant and Young Child.* London: Academia Press, 1970.

10. Kagan, J. and Lewis, M.: Studies of attention in the human infant. *Merrill-Palmer Quarterly,* 1965, *11,* 95-127.

11. Kaplan, Netta R. and Kaplan, Marvin L.: Differential patterns of maternal behavior towards speech defective and non-speech defective children. Proceedings of the 76th Annual Convention, American Psychological Association, San Francisco, 1968.

12. Kenney, E. T.: Mother-retarded child relationships. *American Journal of Mental Deficiency,* 1967, *71* (4), 631-636.

13. Lackner, J. R.: A developmental study of language behavior in retarded children. *Neuropsychologia,* 1968, *6,* 301-320.

14. Lennenberg, Eric H.: *Biological Foundation of Language.* New York: Wiley and Sons, 1967.

15. Lewis, Michael and Freedle, Roy: *Mother-Infant Dyad: The Cradle of Meaning.* Educational Testing Service: Princeton, N. J., 1972.

16. Marshall, N. R., Hegrenes, J. R. and Goldstein, S.: Verbal interactions: Mothers and their retarded children vs. mothers and their non-retarded children. *American Journal of Mental Deficiency,* 1973, *77,* 415-419.

17. Miller, J. and Yoder, D.: An ontogenetic language teaching strategy for retarded children. In Schiefelbusch, R. L. and Lloyd, L. (eds.) *Language Perspectives: Acquisition, Retardation and Intervention.* Baltimore: University Park Press (in press).

18. Minton, C., Kagan, J. and Levine, J.: Maternal control and obedience in the 2-year old. *Child Development,* 1971, *42,* 1873-1894.

19. Moss, H. A.: Sex, age and state as determinants of mother-child interaction. *Merrill-Palmer Quarterly,* 1967, *13,* 19-36.

20. Olim, Ellis G.: Maternal language styles and cognitive development. In Williams, Frederick (ed.) *Language and Poverty,* Chicago: Markham, 1970.

21. Osofsky, J. D. and O'Connell, E. J.: Parent-child interaction: Daughters' effects upon mothers' and fathers' behaviors. *Developmental Psychology,* 1972. *7,* (2), 157-168.

22. Sharlin, S. A. and Polansky, N. A.: The process of infantilization. *American Journal of Orthopsychiatry,* 1972, *42,* 92-102.

23. Siegel, Sidney.: *Nonparametric Statistics for the Behavioral Sciences.* New York: McGraw-Hill, 1956.

24. Snow, Catherine: Mothers' speech to children learning language. *Child Development.* 1972, *43,* 549-565.

25. STAYTON, D. J. HOGAN, R. and AINSWORTH, M. D.: Infant obedience and maternal behavior: The origins of socialization reconsidered. *Child Development,* 1971, *42,* (4), 1057-1069.
26. TERDAL, L. and SEITZ, S.: A group modeling approach to changing parent-child interactions. Paper presented to AAMD Meeting, Minneapolis, May, 1972.
27. THOMAN, E., DENENBERG, V., BECKER, P., GAULIN-KREMER, E., POINDEXTER, M., and SHAW, J.: Analysis of mother-infant interaction sequences: A model for relating mother-infant interactions to the infant's development of behavioral states. Paper presented to Society for Research in Child Development, Philadelphia, March, 1973.
28. TULKIN, STEVEN R. and KAGAN, JEROME: Mother-child interaction in the first year of life. *Child Development,* 1972, *43,* 31-41.
29. WHITEHURST, GROVER J., NOVAK, G., and ZORN, G. A.: Delayed speech studied in the home. *Developmental Psychology,* 1972, *7,* 169-177.

17

Community Attitudes and Down's Syndrome

ROBERT B. EDGERTON, PH.D.

As the care of mentally retarded persons has shifted from large residential facilities to smaller, community-based alternative programs, there has developed a heightened sense of awareness that "community attitudes" are an integral part of a treatment program. Of course, what people think and feel about mental retardation has always been important, whether the people involved are parents of a retarded child, neighbors, social workers, pediatricians, or school teachers. But with a philosophy of normalization now the guiding principle for mental retardation, what members of the community think about mentally retarded persons necessarily takes on primary importance. This paper will briefly 1) review what is known about community attitudes toward mental retardation, 2) discuss the problems involved in determining what are community attitudes, and 3) consider the relevance of community attitudes for research concerning Down's Syndrome.

COMMUNITY ATTITUDES TOWARD MENTAL RETARDATION

Despite the obvious relevance of community attitudes for the treatment of mentally retarded persons, the existing literature on

The research on which this paper was based was supported in part by PHS Grant #HDO4612 NICHD, the Mental Retardation Research Center, U.C.L.A., #HD-05540-02, Patterns of Care and the Development of the Retarded, and 54-71020/9-01, Social Rehabilitation Services.

this subject is strikingly inadequate. The studies which have been published are often both conceptually and methodologically limited, and the findings which have been reported are, perhaps as a consequence, frequently contradictory and difficult to interpret. Since a recent review of this literature is now available (11), I shall only summarize the major findings here.

A large part of the literature deals with parental attitudes, but the findings are varied and conflicting. For example, some studies have reported that the lower the socioeconomic status of the parents of mentally retarded children, the more negative their attitude toward mental retardation, but other studies have reported just the opposite. Other equally conflicting contrasts have also been reported. One of the more consistent findings relates to religion, with Catholic parents being reported, in general, as more accepting of their mentally retarded child than Protestant parents (12). Another large body of research reports the attitudes of institutional employees. Here again attitudes are reported to vary enormously, not only from state to state and institution to institution, but also between wards or programs of a single institution and among individuals within such a ward or program.

Somewhat less diversity is found in the reports about other categories of respondents. Pediatricians, for example, were until recently reported to have generally negative attitudes toward severe mental retardation and to favor institutional rather than home care. Reports over the past five years or so have recorded changes in both of these attitudes. Teachers in both regular and special classes have consistently expressed rather negative attitudes to mentally retarded students, especially to Trainable Mentally Retarded (TMR). It has also been reported with some consistency that teachers are quite susceptible to self-fulfilling prophecies or the so-called Rosenthal effect (19) regarding the intelligence and academic abilities of their students. Whatever consistency may exist in the attitudes of pediatricians or teachers is not reflected in the last major category of this literature—the attitudes of retarded persons themselves. Although compared to non-retarded persons, mentally retarded persons typically express low self-esteem, how much this self-esteem is lowered, and in what ways, vary markedly depending upon such factors as area of the country, severity of the retardation, ethnicity, placement in regular vs. special class, and familial vs. institutional residence.

In this literature about attitudes, one category of persons is seldom represented, namely, the general public. One recent effort to survey such attitudes among differing ethnic groups reported a complex attitudinal pattern. Edgerton and Karno (9) surveyed a probability sample of over 200 Anglo- and 400 Mexican-Americans in East Los Angeles. Each respondent was asked, among other things, about the preferred course of action with regard to family vs. hospital care for a five-year-old TMR boy if the cost of the two forms of care were equal. Both Anglo-American and Mexican-American respondents tended to prefer home care to hospital, but they did so for quite different, and somewhat conflicting, reasons. Furthermore, within each ethnic population there was substantial variation in the attitudes that were expressed. Edgerton and Karno concluded that the presence of such diversity among these low socioeconomic status populations reflected social and motivational complexity, knowledge of which was highly relevant for those who plan and provide services for the mentally retarded.

COMMUNITY ATTITUDES TOWARD DOWN'S SYNDROME

What do we know about "community attitudes" toward Down's Syndrome (DS)? The literature concerning attitudes toward DS children or adults is limited and contains limited empirical data, but these data are reasonably consistent; not much is known, but what is reported by one investigator is usually confirmed by subsequent investigators (e.g., Schipper (20), Kramm (16), Ehlers (10), Jacobs (14), Apgar (1), Share and Landman (23)). Thus, it is generally agreed that the negative attitudes of teachers toward TMR children are extended to DS children, and that pediatricians are often negative about the prospects of DS children, tending, more often than parents like to hear, to favor institutionalization. On the other hand, parents of DS children seem to be more positive in their attitudes than are parents of other TMR children, and siblings of DS children are reported to be more often positive than negative, with the majority said to be understanding and helpful.

Little is known about the attitudes of the general public toward DS persons, but the literature on stereotypic personality among DS persons may provide suggestions about what such an attitude might be. For example, from the earliest days when Down identified the syndrome until quite recently, there have been assertions about the homogeneous character of DS persons. They have been characterized as imitative, cute, musical, harmless, pleasant, and the like. This stereotype has been greatly overdrawn (25) and may, indeed, have no validity whatever (23), but it is nevertheless widespread and could serve to influence public attitudes.

That the existing body of research on community attitudes toward mental retardation is an inadequate basis upon which to plan for the needs of the mentally retarded is an obvious and inescapable conclusion. The available research is fragmentary, rarely cumulative, methodologically naive and lacking articulation to a body of theory. While it is important to recognize the inadequacies of this literature, it is also important to realize that some of the problems inherent in this literature would be troublesome in any organized effort to determine "community attitudes" toward any affliction, disability, or condition.

SOME PROBLEMS IN THE STUDY OF COMMUNITY ATTITUDES

How does one sample attitudes toward mental retardation in a nation as large and heterogeneous as the United States? To investigate even the more superficial nature of regional, religious, class, and ethnic variation in attitudes toward mental retardation would be an enormous undertaking. But even if such an immense enterprise were to be undertaken, how would one cope with the rapid changes that are so much a feature of life in the United States? For example, sexual attitudes are changing so rapidly that few among us have the temerity to guess where they may go next, but fewer still would be foolish enough to believe that they will not continue to change (6). Size, diversity, and change then are formidable obstacles to any effort to assay attitudes in this country, as our large and prosperous opinion polling and survey research organizations have discovered. But these are problems which can be overcome, as the opinion pollsters have done, if enough people representative of the country's relevant diversity are surveyed often enough. Cost is the consideration, and unfortunately it is not as profitable to measure attitudes toward mental retardation as it is to predict voting patterns.

But there are other problems in attitude measurement that are not so easily dealt with. One problem has to do with the concept "community." It is obvious that this concept is meant to embrace a variety of people who fall into certain categories (parent, teacher, doctor, etc.). But it is also used to refer to an actual collectivity of people who live in a geographic area, know their own membership, have some sense of commonality, and so forth. Clearly then, the term embraces even more diversity and change than we have already pointed to. What attitudes does a community *qua* community possess? What about the housewives, grocers, theater owners, mailmen, policemen, and teenagers who make up that community? They may all be part of a local community which helps to shape their attitudes, but they may also have attitudes which are more akin to those held by members of their social category outside their community than to non-members of their category within that community. That is, a policeman in a small Alabama town could be more like a policeman in Cleveland than a grocer in his own small town.

Another problem is the concept "attitude" itself. It is an omnibus term reflecting various cognitive and affective concepts, and hence its referent is sometimes unclear. This is so in the mental retardation literature where the tendency has often been to deal with the cognitive rather than affective components of attitudes. What people think about mental retardation may not be the same as how they *feel*—really feel— about it (5). Another problem is raised by the fact that attitudes can be situation specific. Quite apart from the problems of "set," which have to do with the conditions under which attitudes are elicited (in a test, in an interview, by questionnaire, etc.) or the attributes of the person eliciting them, there are problems brought on by the fact that human behavior and attitudes differ from situation to situation. Consequently, even if an investigator were to correctly discover what attitudes might obtain in one situation, he could not be assured that these same attitudes would obtain in another situation.

But there is a still more basic problem. It is true that what people say in one situation may differ from what they say in another, but whatever it is they say, it may have nothing to do with how they behave. The sociologist Irwin Deutscher (7) has written about the differences between "words" and "deeds," pointing to the extraordinary emphasis in the social sciences upon the study of words, and the remarkable absence of evidence to indicate that one can predict what people will do from a knowledge of what they say.

An illustration is in order. In the early 1930's, the sociologist Richard LaPiere (17) set out to test the relationship of words to deeds, or as he called them, "attitudes" and "actions." Traveling with a Chinese couple who were friends of his, he spent two years crossing the United States and going up and down the West Coast. Those were years of overt public discrimination against Chinese, among other people. Nevertheless, of the 251 hotels and restaurants the Chinese couple visited, only one refused accommodation or service. Puzzled by this result, LaPiere six months later sent a letter to each establishment that he and his friends had visited, asking: "Would you accept members of the Chinese race as guests in your establishment?" Only one letter replied that they would, and this was from a lady who reminisced about the nice Chinese couple she had put up some six months earlier. Thinking that his visit with the Chinese couple may have affected the way that proprietors responded, LaPiere chose a large number of hotels and restaurants which the Chinese couple had not visited but which seemed to be similar to the ones they had visited. The same letter was sent and the responses were the same. Ninety-two percent said they would not accept Chinese, and the remainder were somehow uncertain; none said that he would accept Chinese. Here then we have a dramatic instance of how different expressed attitudes and actual behaviors can be.

As Deutscher (7) and others have pointed out, similar discrepancies have been found in many other studies. The point is not that people never behave as they say they will, but that they very often do not, and that verbal expressions of attitude therefore are an unreliable predictor of behavior.

WORDS, DEEDS, AND THE MENTALLY RETARDED

After 14 years of empirical research with mentally retarded persons and their "communitites" here and abroad, I feel confident in saying that as far as this population is concerned, at least, what people do with regard to them is neither entirely predictable nor comprehensible on the basis of what they say about them. During this period of research, my associates and I have studied large institutions and smaller ones including all the present day versions of alternative residential care, have followed persons released (or escaped) from those places, have spent considerable time with mentally retarded persons in their parents' homes and their own, and have examined the role of mentally retarded persons in Africa and Polynesia.

The attitudinal and behavioral contradictions are always present. For example, among the Pokot of Kenya there are strong cultural attitudes against the survival of retarded persons, yet such persons do survive and are protected, and so it is in many parts of the world (8). Conversely, among Americans whose job it is to care for the retarded, it is common to hear the most pious pronouncements about love, respect, help, and the like, only to discover that talk is indeed cheap and that actual behavior often reveals something considerably less ennobled and humane.

Disillusionments of this sort long ago led anthropologists to develop techniques of fieldwork that relied upon prolonged residence with the persons being studied. After many months of observation, conversation, and participation, usually carried out in the most indirect and unobtrusive ways, an anthropologist *begins* to believe that he understands something about the relationship between behavior and attitudes. After more months he frequently realizes how mistaken he was, and sometimes, but only sometimes, after additional time, he truly begins to understand why people talk and behave in the ways they do. The point—that words are not necessarily the same as deeds—is obvious but it is too seldom taken seriously.

ATTITUDES AND DOWN'S SYNDROME RESEARCH

During my years of research with the mentally retarded I have noticed that more and more DS people are present in public places (restaurants, markets, places of entertainment, buses, etc.) and that other people in these places take less and less notice of the DS people. Usually the DS person is obviously accompanied by someone, but occasionally he or she (usually an adult) is not. I have carried out no systematic research focused upon community attitudes or behaviors toward DS people, but I have recently asked persons in various retail businesses, including restaurants, and persons in mental retardation caretaking roles if they agreed with my observation that DS persons are seen in public more often than they were in the past. Well over 90% of the 50 or so persons questioned throughout the Southern California area agreed that DS people were indeed more visible in public places. This is not offered as a research finding, but merely as a suggestion that something may be changing in the ways that DS persons and members of the general public behave toward one another.

Relatively little is now known about public or community attitudes toward DS persons. A comprehensive body of data about such attitudes in the United States could, presumably, be acquired, but the effort required would be enormous, and the resulting data could be rapidly outdated by social, economic or technological changes. Furthermore, even if community attitudes could be accurately ascertained, the actual behavior of the people in various communities might not be consistent with their expressed attitudes.

Since the principal purpose of research on community attitudes toward DS people would not be theoretical but practical, centering upon facilitation of the normalization process, we should ask what directions such research might most profitably follow. Two directions can be suggested to illustrate the choices that might be made: (1) that a concerted effort be made to create favorable attitudes toward

DS, and, (2) that research focus upon the reciprocal behaviors of DS persons and others in various community settings. A brief discussion of these two kinds of approaches may help to clarify the issues.

First, it should be noted that there is a sizable literature on the theories and methods of attitude change (e.g., Bakan (2); Kiesler, Collins and Miller (15); McGuire (18); Scott (21); and Bem (4)). There is also a considerable body of research relating to changing the attitudes people hold toward mental retardation. In general this research reports that efforts to create more positive attitudes have not been very successful, but that the greatest success seems to come when members of the community are placed in contact with retarded persons and are provided with positive information about them (3, 26). The second approach, which emphasizes behavior, need not rely upon specific forms of behavior theory. It can instead simply study social, legal, or economic changes that in themselves bring about changes in behavior. A dramatic recent example can be taken from the civil rights or Black Power movements. Attitudes may or may not have changed as a result of these social changes, but behaviors have. Whether one derives one's confidence that socioeconomic change can bring about changes in behavior—and eventually in attitudes—from empirical inferences based upon recent social change, or from some version of materialist theory, hardly matters.

If the suggestion made earlier that DS people are increasingly entering into at least some domains of normal community life is correct, then a naturally occurring research opportunity already exists. There is evidence from various sources (including DS parents' groups) that many parents have already gone a long way toward normalizing the home environments of their DS children with resulting improvement in the adaptive behavior of these children (1, 23). Some of these parents are taking their DS children (and adults) more and more into the community where they presumably continue to display the trust, confidence, and love shown in the home. If this behavior does indeed occur, one could hypothesize that members of the community will behave toward the DS person as the members of the family do. Once the behaviors of normalization are established, more positive attitudes may follow. Even if they do not, however, the establishment of more normalized behaviors would seem to be the first concern.

It may well be correct, as various people have suggested (24), that how people think, feel, and behave toward DS people (or other retarded persons) is a function of such factors as the visibility of their affliction, its interference with normal communication, the reversibility of the prognosis, the extent of the behavioral incapacity including difficulties in daily living, and existing social stigma. No doubt these factors, and others, are related to both behaviors and attitudes, but it is by no means clear which, if any, may be causative and which merely epiphenomenal of more fundamental social and cultural considerations (8).

The answers lie in research, of course, but in my opinion, not primarily in research dealing with community attitudes. Instead, I would urge that research examine the interactions between parents (or siblings), the DS person, and community members. These interactions occur throughout the United States in a great variety of settings. By observing how parents and DS persons present and comport themselves in public places and by observing the responses of normal persons, we can unobtrusively determine what the tolerance limits may be for certain kinds of DS persons, accompanied or not, to engage in certain activities in certain kinds of places. Such information, if it were collected, could help parents to know how far they can reasonably go in attempting to provide a normalized community life for their child. While such research is being contemplated, there is one kind of attitude research that is inexpensive, highly informative, and seldom carried out, namely, reporting the attitudes of DS persons themselves. Such persons have much to tell us (13, 22) about themselves and about the communities in which they live.

REFERENCES

1. Apgar, V. (Ed.): Down's Syndrome (mongolism). *Annals of the New York Academy of Sciences*. Vol. 171: 303-688, 1970.
2. Bakan, D.: *On Method: Toward a Reconstruction of Psychological Theory*. San Francisco: Jossey-Bass, 1968.
3. Begab, M. J.: The effect of differences in curricula and experiences on social work student attitudes and knowledge about mental retardation. *Dissertation Abstracts*. 29, (11-A), 4111-4112, 1969.

4. BEM, D. J.: *Beliefs, Attitudes and Human Affairs.* Belmont, California: Brooks/Cole, 1970.
5. CRANDELL, J. M.: The genesis and modification of attitudes toward the child who is different. *Training School Bulletin.* 66: 72-79, 1969.
6. DE LA CRUZ, F. and LAVECK, G. D. (Eds.): *Human Sexuality and the Mentally Retarded.* New York: Brunner/Mazel, 1973.
7. DEUTSCHER, I.: Words and deeds: Social science and social policy. *Social Problems.* 13: 233-254, 1966.
8. EDGERTON, R. B.: Mental retardation in non-western societies: Toward a cross-cultural perspective on incompetence. In H. C. Haywood, Ed., *Social-Cultural Aspects of Mental Retardation.* New York: Appleton-Century-Crofts, pp. 523-559, 1970.
9. EDGERTON, R. B. and KARNO, M.: Community attitudes toward the hospital care of the mentally retarded. *Mental Retardation.* 10: 3-5, 1972.
10. EHLERS, W. H.: *Mothers of Retarded Children: How They Feel, Where They Find Help.* Springfield, Ill.: Charles C. Thomas, 1966.
11. HARTH, R.: Attitudes and mental retardation. Review of the literature. *Training School Bulletin.* 69: 150-164, 1973.
12. HOFFMAN, J. L.: Mental retardation, religious values, and psychiatric universe. *American Journal of Psychiatry.* 121, 885-889, 1965.
13. HUNT, N.: *The World of Nigel Hunt: The Diary of a Mongoloid Youth.* New York: Garrett, 1967.
14. JACOBS, J.: The search for help: A study of the retarded child in the community. New York: Brunner/Mazel, 1969.
15. KIESLER, C. A., COLLINS, B. E., and MILLER, N.: *Attitude Change.* New York: Wiley, 1969.
16. KRAMM, E. R.: *Families of Mongoloid Children.* Washington, D.C.: Children's Bureau, U.S. Department of Health, Education and Welfare, 1963.
17. LAPIERE, R. T.: Attitudes vs. actions. *Social Forces.* 13: 230-237, 1934.
18. MCGUIRE, W. J.: The nature of attitudes and attitude change, In G. Lindzey and E. Aronson, Eds., *The Handbook of Social Psychology,* 2nd Ed. Vol. III. Reading, Mass.: Addison-Wesley, pp. 136-314, 1969.
19. ROSENTHAL, R. and JACOBSON, L.: *Pygmalion in the Classroom.* New. York: Holt, Rinehart & Winston, 1968.
20. SCHIPPER, M. T.: The child with mongolism in the home. *Pediatrics.* 24: 132, 1959.
21. SCOTT, W. A.: Attitude measurement. In G. Lindzey and E. Aronson, Eds., *The Handbook of Social Psychology,* 2nd Ed. Vol I. Reading, Mass.: Addison-Wesley, pp. 204-273, 1969.
22. SEAGOE, V. M.: *Yesterday was Tuesday, All Day and All Night.* Boston: Little, Brown, 1964.
23. SHARE, J. and LANDMAN, G.: Down's Syndrome Longitudinal Study, Technical Report, SERP 1972, A-7, UCLA, pp. 91, Nov. 1972.
24. SHEARS, L. M. and JENSEMA, C. J.: Social acceptability of anomalous. *Exceptional Children.* 35: 91-96, 1969.
25. SILVERSTEIN, A. B.: An empirical test of the mongoloid stereotype. *American Journal of Mental Deficiency.* 68: 493, 1964.
26. STAUCH, J. D.: Social contact as a variable in the expressed attitudes of normal adolescents toward EMR Pupils. *Exceptional Children.* 36, 495-500, 1970.

18

Preparation for Employment

FLOYD R. SWANSON

As Chief of the Personnel Staffing Branch within the Office of Personnel Management of a large government agency, the National Institutes of Health (NIH), my role in this agency is to develop, implement and coordinate a variety of staffing programs, procedures and activities. The NIH is made up of some 19 bureaus, institutes and divisions, and the total employment is approximately 12,000 full-time employees.

My experiences are drawn from the NIH and from the people who work there. In order to develop this chapter, it was necessary to talk with a number of people who have been directly involved with the employment of the mentally retarded. I would like to share with you some of the varied experiences which were related to me, as I had the opportunity to explore a variety of employment situations at the NIH.

I would like to make it clear at the outset that I am drawing upon NIH employment experiences with the mentally retarded and that by and large my experience with those who have Down's Syndrome is quite limited. My opinions are far from scientific. They are observations made from the anecdotal material gathered from several institutes within NIH where the mentally retarded are employed.

Many of us have experienced the difficulties and frustrations of seeking employment with a large Federal agency. You are probably aware, then, of the problems the mentally retarded face in their attempts to enter the world of work in a bureaucracy. It is from my perspective in the bureaucracy that I would like to present to you some experiences involving employment of the retarded. Let us start with Cliff.

CLIFF—A GOOD WORKER

Cliff is a messenger. He delivers the mail for one of the institutes within NIH. He also does a limited amount of xerox work. He has held his job for several years. He is quite well known at NIH by his fellow employees, by virtue of the fact that he sings while making his rounds. He is cheerful, outgoing, and gregarious in his relationships. Most of the people recognize that Cliff is mentally retarded, while only some, I suspect, realize he has Down's Syndrome.

Cliff does a very good job and because of his outgoing nature and his spontaneous singing habits he is a welcome influence on all. Cliff helps to relieve the daily pattern of work, and I find this an extra bonus in addition to the good job he does in delivering the mail.

Cliff is an interesting person and there are many anecdotes about him. Recently, his institute had a birthday party for itself. When Cliff heard they were planning some entertainment and needed volunteers, he volunteered to sing. He delivered a splendid rendition of one of his favorite songs, "16 Tons." And at last year's Christmas Party, Cliff led a group of employees in singing Christmas carols.

Cliff also reads a good deal. He is currently reading the Bible. He has developed a friendship with the director of his institute and he frequently draws books from the library for the director's reading pleasure. I'm told that Cliff personally makes the selection of reading material based on what he thinks the director will like.

Cliff is not always cheerful and agreeable; he can be angry at times. He has his "mad days." He recently announced that he had ". . . done enough for the Institute." Fortunately, Cliff's supervisor knows how to handle him. He lets Cliff blow off steam and soon he is back on the track.

Cliff is very dependable and reliable, takes very little time off and then only when absolutely necessary. Recently, his supervisor got a call from one of the NIH receptionists who saw Cliff outside the building throwing up on the sidewalk. The supervisor rushed down to get Cliff and to help him back into his office. Obviously Cliff was sick and needed attention. Although his illness was not serious, Cliff's concern was in getting the mail out. His supervisor had to patiently convince him that someone else would take care of the mail that day.

Cliff comes to work at 7:00 a.m., 1½ hours before the regular starting time of 8:30 a.m. One morning he was late. It seems he was waiting for the morning paper to be delivered before going to work. This is his routine—first the paper arrives, then he goes to work. It turned out the paper boy did not deliver that morning. Someone from Cliff's office called him and he finally came in to work. It was, nonetheless, a break in his anticipated routine which required, for Cliff, some explanation, and help in getting back into his established pattern. At that time he was living alone. He is now back with his parents. I understand he will be moving in the near future into a supervised group living arrangement for the developmentally handicapped.

A few years ago, Cliff was not always so cheerful when greeted in the corridor while he was making his rounds. It was an interruption of his routine and disturbed his concentration. Now that he has mastered his job, it is no longer a problem for Cliff to be interrupted.

Not long ago Cliff was observed prostrate on the floor of one of the offices where he had been delivering the mail. The rescue squad was quickly called in and he was rushed to the hospital. Everyone thought something serious had happened to Cliff. It turned out, however, that he had simply laid down to relieve a slight dizzy spell. His doctor had told him to lie down whenever he felt dizzy. So he followed his doctor's orders and lay down on the floor of the office exactly where he happened to feel dizzy. That episode caused quite a commotion among Cliff's friends who assumed something dreadful had happened. Cliff, however, was back on the job the next day.

As we noted earlier, Cliff is a very interesting person and a good employee of the NIH. He is a reliable, dependable and competent worker. And, with his uninhibited singing, he brightens our day.

MARTHA—DEALING WITH HIDDEN PROBLEMS

Let's look at Martha, another NIH employee who is mentally retarded. Her job is in another Institute and it is a messenger position much like Cliff's. Martha had hidden problems that did not immediately manifest themselves, but when they did they required a patient and sympathetic supervisor.

Martha was referred to NIH by a state vocational rehabilitation service. We should note here that Federal agencies are provided a special appointing authority for the mentally retarded. This "excepted" authority may only be used for persons who are evaluated and certified by state vocational rehabilitation services. All of the examples I cite have been appointed under this special authority. I might also add that persons employed under this authority enjoy the coverage of group life and health insurance, annual leave and other benefits afforded all employees.

Martha was referred from the state vocational rehabilitation service and she was accompanied by her counselor. She was interviewed by personnel specialists and by a supervisor who had employed several other persons who were also mentally retarded. Martha was selected for the job.

It seems that Martha was not learning her duties as well or as quickly as expected. Her supervisor knew she was retarded, but based on his experience with other retarded employees he felt she should be doing better. He talked with Martha and noticed that her glasses had a hearing aid built into them. Since Martha wore her glasses only occasionally, it became apparent that she was hearing instructions only part of the time. Once this was discovered, it was easy to insure that Martha was hearing instructions from then on. She was told to wear her glasses, and then she was told what her duties and responsibilities would be.

Martha had a seizure one day. Her supervisor discovered she had epilepsy, for which she was taking medication. While this did not interfere with her work in any continuing way, it was another hidden problem which had not been brought to her supervisor's attention at the time of employment.

Martha also had an active social life which turned out to be another on-the-job problem. She was attractive and had boyfriends. Her supervisor found out that she was having sexual relations at work which had become well known among the work force.

The supervisor sought advice from her counselor and also brought the situation to the attention of Martha's parents. He was able to get little or no help from these sources. He finally talked to her directly, telling her that her conduct was not acceptable, that it would have to change or she would be fired.

Apparently this stern and candid talk with Martha corrected her on-the-job behavior, and she has become a reliable and dependable employee with no more sex on the job.

The employment of Cliff and Martha demonstrates the importance of good supervision toward the successful adjustment of the retarded to their work environment.

ALICE—THE SUPERVISOR'S ROLE

The supervisor's role is crucial in the placement of the retarded. The supervisor of an employee named Alice tells how she resented, at first, being asked to even consider employment of someone who was retarded. This supervisor had a very heavy work load directing the activities of a Grants and Contracts Section and she frankly did not see how a retarded person could help out.

Nevertheless, she did accept Alice's placement in her section and set about establishing a pattern of work which Alice could perform. At first the supervisor found Alice withdrawn and seemingly disinterested. It took some time to overcome these initial barriers. As her supervisor got to know Alice, it became apparent that she was interested in her work and that she could do it well.

The supervisor also found that there was some resentment and misunderstanding among Alice's fellow employees. Through discussion with other employees in the section, the supervisor was able to develop a greater understanding and empathy on the part of these employees toward Alice. Soon a better working climate for Alice was established.

Under these positive conditions, Alice prospered. She became a very good employee and she began to develop her own friendships among those she met at work. She was able to assume a variety of tasks such as collating, labeling, stapling, simple filing and messenger work.

One day Alice discovered an error in labeling of some study section books which she was collating. This involved the dates of some meetings which if not corrected would have brought some of the Institute consultants in from out of town on the wrong dates. Alice's supervisor was naturally most gratified with Alice's alertness in noticing the mix-up of dates. She praised Alice for bringing this error to her attention. Alice, who recognized that her discovery was very important, took a great deal of pride and satisfaction in having found the error.

Alice has worked at NIH for four years. She has been promoted and she has received a "quality step increase" in salary. The citation for Alice's quality increase reads in part ". . . In the overall execution of her duties, she has shown a remarkable degree of energy and industry . . . [she] works efficiently and accurately in handling an unusually large volume of routine work. . ."

Alice's story is instructive, I think, because it represents her success and also the success of her supervisor in helping Alice to become a good employee.

PETER, PAUL AND PHIL—COMPLEX ADJUSTMENT PROBLEMS

I would like to shift our focus to another Institute within NIH where management made a decision, a little over a year ago, to set aside three openings for employment of the retarded. This example differs from the others I have cited in that management recognized that the mentally retarded might be useful in certain kinds of jobs and took steps to seek out candidates. I should point out that the Institute where Martha, whom we discussed earlier, works does employ several mentally retarded persons and initiated their employment practices several years earlier.

The three jobs established by the new Institute taking the plunge with employment of the retarded were in the area of animal caretaking, involving cage washing, glassware washing and the like. Let's call the candidates for the three jobs Peter, Paul, and Phil.

Management officials of the Institute worked closely with their personnel officer and with the state vocational rehabilitation people in the interviewing and selection process. The job requirements were reviewed by the vocational counselors and Peter, Paul and Phil were presented as candidates for the positions. The supervisors also spent some time preparing other employees already in the section for the prospect of employment of the retarded.

The time spent talking with other employees and preparing them for the employment of co-workers who would be retarded was well spent. It was found that the regular employees were threatened to some extent by the prospect of the hiring of the retarded. They felt that somehow the retarded might be given preferential treatment with regard to promotion. This fear was dispelled when it was explained that the retarded employees could expect only limited advancement at least in keeping with their job skills. In fact, it was likely that the regular employees could expect greater advancement possibilities, since they would be free to assume higher level responsibilities.

Of the three, Peter proved to be an excellent employee. His supervisor had good success with him and several follow-up visits by his counselor provided the necessary support toward Peter's work adjustment.

Paul and Phil, however, developed an antagonistic relationship toward each other. Paul, it seems, was somewhat of a bully toward Phil. Phil complained and their counselors were brought in to help analyze and, hopefully, resolve the situation. Their problems were not successfully resolved. Phil began taking more and more time off from the job, and he also became increasingly fretful about " . . . missing work and letting people down." He finally resigned.

Paul found himself in some difficulty with other employees, who would come to Phil's defense. These conflicts were eventually worked out, and, at this juncture, Paul has made a fairly good adjustment and is expected to continue on in his work.

The employment of Peter, Paul and Phil illustrates more complex adjustment problems. In working toward their placement and in understanding some of their problems, the involvement of the vocational counselor was most valuable. The counselor was helpful in every step of the placement process and during the follow-up sessions. Although Phil's employment did not work out, the employment of the others has. The management officials of this Institute, who made a commitment to employ the mentally retarded, followed through with it and they will be hiring more.

ROLES OF COUNSELORS, SUPERVISORS, AND MANAGEMENT

The examples I have given are but a few of the 32 mentally retarded persons currently employed by the NIH. As we observed earlier, finding a job in a large bureaucracy can be an imposing task. The employment of the retarded is dependent on those people involved in the process: the vocational rehabilitation counselors, the personnel specialist, the supervisor, and management.

I think the role of the counselor is very important, especially in the initial stages of interviewing and placement and during the first few weeks on the job. The NIH experiences do not, however, indicate that the counselor is always helpful or has a positive effect. For example, in the case of Alice, there was a reorganization in her Institute, and she was going to have to move to a new office. Since this would involve a new assignment, her counselor was asked to assist in helping her make the adjustment. It turned out that he was not particularly sensitive to the situation and he caused Alice to become quite upset about the change in assignments. Fortunately, Alice's supervisor was able to calm her and the reassignment was finally worked out. I might add that a small change of work assignments can be stimulating to the employee.

The counselor's role in helping Martha, who had a variety of problems, was also of little value. Again, it was Martha's supervisor who through his patience and firmness was able to deal with her problems and resolve them.

In the majority of cases, we have found the counselor to be most helpful and sensitive in the preparation for employment. The counselor is always part of the process and usually a strong, positive influence.

The supervisor's role is critical, and, I think, the key to a good work adjustment on the part of the retarded. A person who agrees to supervise someone who is retarded must be patient and firm. A supervisor who can't exercise discipline and command the respect of his employees is not likely to do well with a retarded employee. Supervisors who employ the retarded must be secure in their own jobs and be able to accept unusual behavior at times. Supervisors who have work suitable for the skills of the retarded have found such employees to be valuable members of the work force.

Management working through personnel specialists and with supervisors can prepare the way for employment of the developmentally handicapped. In these times an organization often finds itself committed to a variety of employment programs: Equal Employment Opportunity, veterans reemployment, employment of women, upward mobility efforts, hiring the handicapped, etc. Those of us involved in staffing often wonder what new program will arrive tomorrow. At NIH the employment of the retarded has often been found to free other employees from routine tasks, permitting them to move toward higher level jobs and advancement. So we see that while some of the special interest employment programs are competitive with one another, the employment of the retarded tends to free people for other work.

As we have had the opportunity to work with the retarded, we have learned much about their capabilities and the contributions they can make to our lives.

The NIH experience with employment of the retarded clearly shows us they are good employees. Through this experience we are given a greater perspective and understanding of the range of human capabilities.

19

Mobility Training for the Retarded

PAT DEL MONICO, M.S.W.

Our ability to be independently mobile opens up a wide range of choices for vocational, educational, recreational, and social activities which would otherwise be seriously limited. And it is largely the availability of alternatives and the opportunity for decision-making that determines the quality of our lives. It is our responsibility, then, to help the retarded to develop the tools they need to be in a position to make some choices about the quality of their lives. We do not choose our friends, our jobs, and our leisure time activities based solely upon their geographic desirability. That would be an unnecessary imposition. And it is unfair to assume that it is not an imposition for the retarded. The fact is that nearly all of the mildly retarded and most of the moderately retarded can be trained to use, effectively and independently, public transportation.

CONQUERING FEARS

There is no question but that there are some very real apprehensions on the part of mentally retarded persons and their parents when considering independent mobility, especially in large impersonal urban settings. The fact that these fears exist is the very reason that their elements must be dealt with rather than disguised or ignored. And it is because of the reality of these fears that mobility training begins in the home and in the classroom and must remain there for several months, perhaps longer.

The mentally retarded adults I have worked with have mentioned consistently two primary fears they have when contemplating traveling about the community alone. Their first trepidation is that they will be recognized as "different" and, as a result, be sneered at or made fun of. Some mentally retarded people have facial stigmata and other physical characteristics which are atypical. In most cases we cannot change these features. We can, however, help them to dress in a manner which is appropriate for their age and in a fashion which is in keeping with the style of the day. There is no more excuse for the mentally retarded person to be seriously obese, or to have unsightly acne, or to be unclean or unkempt than there is for a typical person to display the same kind of personal disregard. We can help the mentally retarded person to take pride in his appearance and thereby lessen the possibility of his being jeered at because of "otherness."

The second fear mentioned by both the mentally retarded trainee and his parents is that he will get lost. The fear of getting lost is dealt with by giving the trainee the tools to get found. When possible the trainee should be taught to recite his name, address, and telephone number. He should carry with him at all times an identification card. The card should contain the typical identifying information and must *not* be used to label the bearer as mentally retarded. He should be taught where to find public telephones (department stores, gas stations, etc.) and how to use them. He should be taught whom to ask for help (policemen, bus drivers, etc.).

Parents are particularly concerned that their retarded children will be taken advantage of by strangers with questionable characters and motivations. The only way to prepare the trainee for such circumstances is to discuss openly the possible dangers of interacting with strangers and to caution him vigorously against it. Role-playing such situations as being offered a ride by a stranger is useful and teaches the correct response.

Parents are often fearful that their retarded child will be physically harmed or injured due to his inability to recognize safety signs and safety hazards. The retarded must be taught, through a series of comprehensive and repetitive educational sessions, to be alert to such signs. Emphasis should be placed on word recognition and the correct response to words such as "danger," "stop," "do not enter," "inflammable," "railroad crossing," "step down," etc. The mobility trainer may wish to take a small group of trainees for walks in the community to point out safety signs and to demonstrate appropriate responses to them.

Total safety can never be completely assured. Each day as we get into our car, light a match, cross a street, or even take a bath we are taking a safety risk. But we do not allow the dangers inherent in everyday living to restrict our activities. So, we must give the retarded the tools to deal with everyday dangers. We must allow them the dignity of risk-taking in the hopes that what results will improve the quality of their everyday existence.

PRACTICING MOBILITY

After the trainee is prepared for coping with safety elements, it is time to begin actual mobility training. The initial stages of practical training also take place in the classroom and on small group field trips. One of the first steps is to familiarize the trainee with the actual vehicle of transportation. In Los Angeles the municipal bus companies have been extremely cooperative. On numerous occasions they have welcomed the trainer and several trainees to visit the lot where the vehicles are parked. Trainees have been able to simulate actual boarding, seating, and disembarking procedures in the parked vehicle. Most public transportation companies have community relations departments which can make arrangements for such visits on a regular basis. In addition, they are usually willing to loan out materials which can be used for mobility instruction.

When the trainee is ready for practical instruction, it *must* be done on a one-to-one basis. This is so for several reasons: (1) groups call attention to themselves and emphasize "otherness," thereby causing the trainees to feel self-conscious; (2) the trainer cannot be certain whether each trainee in the group is actually learning the procedure or following the others; (3) the trainees' points of origin (their homes) are usually different and this can cause considerable confusion.

A trainee must always be instructed with a specific destination in mind. Training begins from the point of origin to and from that destination and that destination *only* until the trainee is able to complete the journey on his own. The point of origin is almost always his place of residence. The destination is always a place of his own choice. Allowing for his own choice increases the possibility of success because of the motivation factor. Destinations chosen usually fall into the following categories: (1) a sheltered workshop or other place of employment; (2) a school or vocational training facility; (3) the home of a friend; (4) the home of a relative; (5) a public recreational area or facility.

One round trip per day at least three days per week should be completed. Initially, the trainer will lead and the trainee will follow his actions. While riding in the vehicle the trainer should point out landmarks and teach the trainee to remain alert at all times. It is most helpful if the trainee can read, but it is *not* necessary—environmental landmarks are often better indicators than street signs. Eventually the trainer will allow the trainee to lead. And, finally, the trainee will complete a round-trip on his own while the trainer follows the vehicle by car.

For best results with maximum reinforcement, the destination should be reachable without the necessity to transfer vehicles. If a transfer is necessary the training should take place from the point of origin to the point of transfer until that much is mastered. Training begins again from the point of transfer to the destination until mastered. And then the two steps are combined until mastered.

As is the case with most learning experiences, transfer of knowledge facilitates the procedure when it is reapplied. And so it may take half as long, or less, to teach the trainee how to reach a second destination.

CONSIDERING OTHER MEANS OF ACHIEVING MOBILITY

In cities or towns where public transportation is either limited or unavailable, we must consider other means of achieving mobility.

In most countries of the world, the two-wheeled bicycle is employed as a means of transportation. As a matter of fact, the United

States, almost exclusively of any other country, views the bicycle as a recreational vehicle to be used primarily by the younger generation. If we can overcome this stigma, the bicycle can be used as an effective means for achieving mobility, particularly in rural settings.

Most moderately retarded individuals who are free of physical handicaps are perfectly capable of learning how to ride a bicycle. Bicycle safety can be taught with the aid of films and other materials easily obtainable through such resources as public libraries or recreational facilities. In many communities the police departments have developed bicycle safety demonstrations and are eager to be called upon for assistance.

For the mildly retarded, whose primary problem is academic retardation and whose judgment can be relied upon, we must not rule out achieving mobility through the use of the automobile. I am presently working with a group of 25 mildly retarded young adults, two of whom have obtained California drivers' licenses. Those of us who work with the retarded in the State of California are aware that it is not necessary to be able to read or write in order to pass the written portion of the drivers' examination. This portion can be administered orally. All that is required are the correct responses to the test items and the ability to recognize and interpret traffic signals and signs.

If you reside in a state where the vehicle code is not flexible in the above described manner, you may wish to advocate for such progressive changes in the law. Vehicle codes which require written examinations discriminate not only against mildly retarded citizens, but also against typical citizens who may be illiterate or foreign speaking.

FINDING THE FINANCIAL RESOURCES FOR MOBILITY TRAINING

Doubtless, mobility training can be a costly service, but finding the financial resources needed to provide this service should not be extraordinarily difficult.

In California public education for the trainable mentally retarded is mandated by law. Because there is not a sufficient number of trainable mentally retarded children to warrant a special class in every school, special schools or classes are located at strategic points and the children are bussed to and from these schools daily, every day for 12 to 15 years of public education. The cost of providing this service is great and extremely limited, at best, in educational value. I suggest that the public schools incorporate mobility training into the curriculum for the trainable mentally retarded beginning at the age of 12. I submit that many of these children will be independently mobile by the age of 15 or 16 years. The schools will save the cost of transporting these individuals for their remaining years of public education and, more significantly, the students will have been taught an invaluable skill.

In California the State Department of Rehabilitation often subsidizes the cost of mobility training for a blind person when it is believed that this skill will enable him to obtain employment, thereby reducing his dependence on the tax dollar for income maintenance. I see no reason why the same philosophy should not be applied to mentally retarded clients of that agency. A significant number of mildly retarded and many moderately retarded individuals could maintain jobs in the competitive work market if job sites were accessible.

In California the Regional Center for the Mentally Retarded subsidizes the cost of private transportation provided by sheltered workshops and activity centers for hundreds of adult mentally retarded clients. The cost of subsidizing this service, in addition to workshop and activity center fees, seriously limits the number of clients who can be so assisted. I submit that the Regional Center dollar would be better spent in training the client to be independently mobile to and from the workshop or activity center. This method would free that agency from at least one type of long-term encumbrance and, consequently, would allow for a greater turnover of recipients of service.

In California there is a major emphasis on providing services for mentally retarded people in the community rather than the State Hospital. The theory is that, in addition to being able to provide a more normal environment, there would be some financial savings as the cost of maintaining large institutions is considerable. One of the arguments against this trend is that services to the retarded in the community are not as conveniently located as they are at the State Hospital. The argument of accessibility to community programs would not be substantiated if mobility training were provided each patient capable of such training upon placement in the community.

There are countless other ways to find the financial resources needed for mobility training. Consider, for example, the fact that many special interest groups are provided services under the aegis of adult education. A case in point is the English-as-a-second-language course offered for foreign visitors and residents in our country. Another case in point is the special course leading to a secondary diploma offered to former high school dropouts. Even the Federal Government has developed educational and vocational training programs for special interest groups. I refer to such programs as the Neighborhood Youth Corps and the Job Corps, both designed to provide for the educational and vocational needs of culturally and environmentally disadvantaged youth.

We must not allow the argument of insufficient funds to restrict our efforts to obtain those services which will enhance the lives of the mentally retarded with whom we are concerned. If we are persistent and creative in our efforts to tap the appropriate resources, the finances needed for mobility training will be made available.

CONCLUSION

In conclusion let me point out that I am aware that the development of the skill of mobility may appear low on the list of priority needs for the retarded. And there is no question that is is one of the least dramatic of controversial issues in the field. However, I am convinced that this is a superficial viewpoint in light of my experience in working with the retarded. I have, in fact, seen that it is the lack of mobility that has contributed, either directly or indirectly, to extreme loneliness and isolation for far too many mentally retarded individuals. And, in American society today, there are few things more profoundly agonizing than loneliness and isolation.

Recently we, in the field of mental retardation, have become enlightened. We have come to see and believe that mentally retarded individuals have civil rights—the right to treatment, the right to education, the right to vote, and in some states the right to marry and have children. We must realize, however, that there are some *human* rights which cannot be legislated. And in our technological society mobility must be considered a human right, for it allows us choice of where and with whom we will live, work, and play. Those among us who are not allowed such choices are totally dependent on others to determine the quality of their lives. I am convinced that it is not necessary for us to continue to foster such dependency.

20

Sexuality in the Mentally Retarded

JOAN ELL, M.S.W.

The mentally retarded, like all humans, are sexual beings. They develop love for self and love for others and they develop sexual energies and feelings which must be understood, accepted, and channeled into socially accepted behavior.

Sexuality is a broad area with dimensions as diverse and as complex as are all the unique qualities of the individuals we serve. We will attempt to answer in general terms the five questions most often asked by parents and professionals.

1. Who among the retarded has sexual needs?
2. When is sexuality expressed?
3. Where should sexuality be expressed?
4. Why has the subject been avoided?
5. How do we provide help and guidance in dealing with sexual problems?

WHO AMONG THE RETARDED HAS SEXUAL NEEDS?

As an intricate component of the human personality, sexuality in its broadest application applies to all persons and, therefore, to all mentally retarded persons. Like others, the mentally retarded have been exposed to external sexual messages and attitudes and internal feelings and experiences. Like others, the intensity and sexual drive vary greatly among retarded individuals. While there is little definitive data available, many people feel that the Down's Syndrome individual has great need for love, touch, and affection, but may in general have a somewhat depressed interest in sexual intercourse. Like others, the way in which sexual expression occurs among the retarded will vary greatly with sociocultural background, religious training, type of living situation, and attitudes of families, teachers, and friends. Like others, sexual expression will occur in various forms and at various times, and, like others, sexuality can lead to fulfillment and life enrichment or it can be a source of frustration and discontent. If we can accept that sexual drives are natural, we can take responsibility for helping the retarded to channel these drives into socially acceptable behavior. We can help the retarded to develop constructive attitudes about sex and if and when relationships of a sexual nature develop, we can provide guidance and supervision so that responsibility joins with opportunity, guidance with human rights, and common sense with idealism. Our first question, who among the retarded has sexual needs, is relatively simple to answer, though the answer may be disquieting. They all do.

WHEN IS SEXUALITY EXPRESSED?

Freud believed that sexuality began with birth, though this theory is not necessarily accepted today. For our purposes, it suffices to state that the development of the mentally retarded child proceeds generally along the normal schedule though more time between stages may be required because of decreased capacities, lowered ability to tolerate stress, and poorer relationships within his world. Babies enjoy touch. They learn to love others. They feel needs and fulfillment of needs. Retarded babies have the same experiences and learn, however slowly, to explore, to manipulate, to love, and to desire love.

During the childhood years new social experience and social learning occur. Wolf whistles, dirty words, pictures hidden in the dresser drawers, suggestive movie lines, secreted objects of strange shape and questionable function, and old wives tales abound. Retarded children hear and see with the same confusion and fascination you and I did. The fairy tales have not changed—the horrors of blindness, insanity or worse following masturbation, stories about storks and cabbage patches, and watermelon seeds. The normal child has far more opportunity for receiving valid information and for social experimentation than do most retarded children. The sexual isolation so often seen in adult mentally retarded persons is formed early and reinforced over time, often leading to inappropriate sexual behavior or repression of sexuality. Children masturbate. They explore their own and other bodies. They use words for shock value. Retarded children do the same things. These are normal expressions of childhood sexuality.

Adolescence brings mob control. The retarded adolescent wants what all teenagers want—to dress in the uniform of the day, to talk on the phone, to go to parties, to shave, to wear false eyelashes. Menstruation begins, breasts develop, hair grows, pimples appear. Nocturnal emissions, unexpected erections, unpredictable tears and anger are shared by normal and retarded adolescents. The retarded person needs more, but usually gets less help with experiences that can be exciting if accepted and understood, or frightening if ignored or punished.

During adolescence and young adulthood some retarded persons advance to interest in sex. Others never progress beyond handholding or picture carrying. All need relationships at some level.

WHERE DOES SEXUALITY HAPPEN?

Sexuality occurs with growth; behavior defined as problematical can happen at home, at school, in the park, at the store. Retarded children need to know that behavior that is allowed in the bedroom is not to be tolerated at the dinner table. The bathroom is not the same as the living room or the school room or the bowling alley. There are few retarded young people who cannot learn to make these distinctions. There are many parents and teachers who do not believe they can be taught and have not attempted to provide the training.

WHY HAS THE SUBJECT BEEN AVOIDED?

We do not need to ask why sexuality is expressed. It is expressed because it exists. We do need to ask why the fact of sexuality in the retarded has not been confronted and why it must be, if the reaching of highest human potential is to be seen as a goal for this group. The area has been avoided for three reasons, the first of which has little to do with the mentally retarded. Sex is controversial in that it incorporates unresolved value questions—questions of morality, religion, and life-style. When we consider the problems of bringing sex education into the curricula for normal children it is little wonder that almost no guidance is given the retarded. When we review sex training materials available to the general public we read vague abstractions expressed in impersonal clinical language illustrated by drawings of "human plumbing." It is little wonder that there is a paucity of material adequately concrete and descriptive for our population. The degree to which our society gains comfort with the topic of sexuality will continue to determine the ease with which we can deal with the sexuality of any particular group.

The second reason why the subject of sex in the retarded has been avoided concerns our failure to accept the fact that children become adults. We view the mentally retarded person as an eternal child, a being without physiological maturity or adult needs. In our residential facilities residents of middle age are referred to as boys and girls. Many agencies serving adults incorporate the word "children" in their titles, as do many parent associations. Infantilized behavior and appearance are encouraged and reinforced. Often groups of retarded persons on outings are particularly noticeable because of hair ribbons, bobby socks, hair styles, and clothing ordinarily worn by children. We need to accept the fact that most mentally retarded persons, even those with extremely limited intellectual functioning, develop adult physiology, adult needs and adult attitudes.

The third reason for avoiding the fact of sexuality in the retarded lies in our inability to distinguish sex from marriage and childbearing. Some mentally retarded persons marry, and some have children, but sexuality does not arise magically at the conclusion of a legal ceremony nor does sexuality equal parenthood. The mentally retarded should have access to all the contraception choices available to us all and should participate in a choice consistent with their personal value system.

Certainly, if we are to provide responsible guidance, we must consider the needs of children born to the retarded as well as the needs of the potential parents. However, the risk of pregnancy in and of itself does not preclude the experiencing of love, relationship, and intimacy to a degree consistent with the development of the individual. Fear of pregnancy does not justify prohibiting dating, or exchanging pictures, or holding hands. It does not justify prohibiting marriage for those few whose ability to relate advances to the degree that marriage may be possible. The possibility of pregnancy must, however, be considered in terms of appropriate supervision. The retarded have a right to freedom from unwanted pregnancy equal to our own.

Few Down's Syndrome persons marry and few have children, but many have sexual needs. As part of our evaluation of the individual, we must assess these needs and provide guidance. And because we have not shed the remnants of our puritanical heritage, because we view the retarded as eternal children, and because we fail to distinguish sex from marriage and parenthood, we have just begun to deal with the question of sexuality. This leads to our final question—HOW?

HOW DO WE RECOGNIZE SEXUALITY?

How do we give instruction and guidance? There are general guidelines for providing information appropriately. Questions should be answered when they are asked. Information should be presented clearly and simply. Information should be presented in common, accepted language without shock and instruction about appropriate words should be given. Help should be sought from professionals and friends who are comfortable with this material. Opportunities of a social nature should be provided and encouraged. Inappropriate sexual behavior must not be tolerated any more than is any other inappropriate behavior. When sexual behavior occurs we must remember that it is not new; we saw it in our normal children and, if we are honest, in ourselves. We must help the retarded to develop pride in their bodies through pleasing appearance and manner. We must support the concept of human rights. The right to express sexuality is equal to the right to express no sexuality. We cannot expect maturity until it occurs, nor can we deny it when it becomes manifest. We must simply accept the sexuality of the mentally retarded person to the degree it is expressed just as we do his intellectual development, his social development, his creativity, and any other component of his personality.

APPENDIX

The Role of the National Association for Retarded Citizens in Developing Research in Mental Retardation

FRANK J. MENOLASCINO, M.D., *and*
LAIRD W. HEAL, PH.D.

Today I want to review the role of the National Association oı Retarded Citizens in stimulating the growth of knowledge about mental retardation. This story is one of the development of the NARC research program and the simultaneous growth of federal research support on behalf of our mentally retarded citizens, including those special ones who have been identified with Down's Syndrome.

The September, 1973 issue of *Mental Retardation News* (1) has the headline, "Redirected Research Program Underway." This headline documents the successful rejuvenation of NARC's own research program. Before describing this redirected research program, some historical perspectives may be helpful.

RESEARCH IN MENTAL RETARDATION BEFORE NARC

When NARC was founded in 1950, there was no national program of research to confront the problems of mental retardation (2). Some dedicated scientists, with little or no financial support, were conducting research in institutions across the country. Some university people, especially in special education departments, were addressing problems involved with the identification and training of mentally retarded children in the classroom. Indeed, the Bureau of the Census had included mental handicap as a special category since 1840 and had typically included data on mentally handicapped individuals in its ten-year reports (3).

During the early 1900's a number of highly regarded scientists and humanitarians (e.g., Wallen, Doll, Goddard, and others) had mounted several projects dealing with psychological and educational problems of mentally retarded citizens. While medical research was largely neglected, one giant stands out from the field—Dr. George Jervis of Letchworth Village in New York became well known for his brilliant work in phenylketonuria and a variety of pathological conditions associated with mental retardation. However, the depression and the second World War in tandem seemed to destroy the momentum built up by these pioneers, and research on behalf of our retarded citizens languished during the second quarter of this century (4).

After World War II, in 1946, the National Mental Health Act resulted in the establishment of two very important institutes. The National Institute of Mental Health (NIMH) and the National Institute of Neurological Diseases and Blindness (NINDB, later NINDS) were to become cornerstones of the tower of knowledge about mental retardation, even though mental retardation was not mentioned in the legislation that established them.

THE FOUNDING AND EARLY DEVELOPMENT OF NARC'S RESEARCH PROGRAM

In 1950, the National Association for Retarded Children, on the occasion of its founding, adopted, as the second of its eight purposes, a commitment, "To further the advancement of ameliorative and preventive study and research in the field of mental retardation and of therapy" (5).

NARC began at once to implement this purpose. Mrs. Lenore Davidson was elected Research Chairman, and she immediately sought the counsel of Dr. Grover Powers (6), who was about to retire after 25 years as the very distinguished Chairman of the

Department of Pediatrics at the Yale University College of Medicine. The NARC Board authorized the selection of the Scientific Research Advisory Board not to exceed 25 members (6), and Dr. Powers was to remain chairman of this Board until 1961.

The state of our knowledge about mental retardation at the time that Dr. Powers took up his challenge is exemplified by a report on an Institute on Mongolism in 1953. This institute was funded by the New York Association for the Help of Retarded Children and the Division of Pediatric Psychiatry at the Brooklyn Jewish Hospital. Dr. T. H. Ingalls of the Harvard School of Public Health, in discussing the prevention and causes of mongolism, stated, "New interpretations of evidence lead us to believe that mongolism has its origin in some damage done to the baby during the first weeks of his life in the mother's womb as the result of numerous factors which seem to occur in mothers who have had many children, or who after a lapse of several years of a parent's sterility conceive in the later child-bearing years, or in many instances after entering the menopause" (8). We have come a long way in 20 years!

NARC SURVEY OF RESEARCH

Dr. Powers felt that the first need of any research program in mental retardation was to survey all that was currently known about mental retardation and then, on the basis of the survey, develop appropriate priorities. In December of 1954, the first Research Advisory Board was announced (9). It consisted of 21 outstanding scientists and educators, including Dr. Samuel Kirk, Dr. Edith Potter, Dr. Seymour Sarason, Dr. Abner Wolf, Dr. Herman Yannet and Dr. George Jervis (who remains on the NARC Research Advisory Committee today). At the same time, Dr. Powers announced the appointment of Dr. Richard Lambert Masland as the Research Survey Director (10). Dr. Masland was then the Associate Professor in charge of Neurology at the Bowman-Gray School of Medicine in Winston-Salem, North Carolina. He was later to become a very influential extension of NARC's contribution to federal research, as the director of the National Institute of Neurological Diseases and Blindness. It was the conviction of both Drs. Powers and Masland that the general research survey on mental retardation should include behavioral, as well as biomedical, research. They therefore recommended that a behavioral scientist be employed to assist with the survey. In 1955 they obtained federal grants from NIMH totalling nearly $50,000 to support their convictions. These grants allowed Dr. Masland to enlist as colleagues Dr. Seymour Sarason, a psychologist from Yale University, and Dr. Thomas Gladwin, an anthropologist with the National Institute of Mental Health. After four years of collation, review, and analysis of the world literature in mental retardation, these men published the classic work, *Mental Subnormality,* in 1958 (11).

The competence and vision of these men are apparent from the conclusions that they drew in this book (12).

Dr. Masland pointed out that there are generally two classes of mentally retarded individuals. Members of the first class, usually of borderline or mild intelligence, are most frequently noted to be handicapped from environmental factors. This group was the one addressed by Sarason and Gladwin. The other group, who appeared to have some damage or injury to the central nervous system, appeared to be mentally retarded for one of four reasons, all of which were amenable to biomedical research: 1) genetic defects; 2) prenatal toxicity; 3) injury to the nervous system occurring near the time of birth; and 4) injury to the nervous system following diseases of childhood and infancy.

In the area of cultural-familial mental retardation, Drs. Sarason and Gladwin (13) recommended research on the following topics:

1. Subcultures within our main culture which provide a child with intellectual training that handicaps him when he must take his place in the larger society;
2. Longitudinal studies to determine the extent to which an individual's intelligence changes over time;
3. Cross-cultural studies in pathology to determine the ways that different cultures give rise to different types of mental retardation;
4. The development of a theory of intelligence including the development of measures of adaptive behavior that are not based on standard school testing and school situations;

5. The study of the relationship between psychosis and mental subnormality;
6. The study of variations in early temperament and their influence on intellectual growth;
7. The recruitment and training of research personnel. Sarason and Gladwin concluded that unless well-trained scientists were attracted to the problems of mental retardation, there could be no successful research on those problems.

With the completion of the survey, which was published by Basic Books and was excerpted in several scholarly publications, the Research Advisory Board began to financially support the research of qualified scientists in university centers.

In the July, 1958 issue of *Mental Retardation News* (14), NARC announced it would support research in four priority areas: "1) Research in the causes, prevention and treatment of mental retardation; 2) Research in accurate evaluation, mental, physical, emotional and social; 3) Research to develop effective training techniques so the mentally retarded can develop their fullest potentialities; 4) Research to find the best framework for living where the mentally retarded can be taught, trained and can work."

The primary emphasis was placed on the biological sciences. Furthermore, Dr. Powers noted, "basic research in the biological sciences can best be encouraged through long-term support of senior investigators or research professorships. . . . NARC's research program thus seeks to ensure that gifted investigators whose scientific interest in mental retardation has been aroused shall be enabled to pursue these interests intensively on a career basis" (15). We shall see that it was this commitment to long-term sustaining grants that drained the vigor of the NARC research program and eventually became one of the seeds of the redirection of 1971. NARC also announced that grants would be made to support symposia or conferences on scientific subjects directly related to mental retardation.

EXPANSION OF FEDERAL PROGRAMS

Simultaneous with the development of the NARC research program was the acceleration of effort and resources committed to mental retardation by the federal government. In 1954, the National Institute of Mental Health awarded a three-year grant of over $122,000 to George Peabody College for the training of research scientists in mental retardation at the doctoral level (16). This program was phenomenally successful and was to become the model for many research training programs funded during the 1960's.

The research thrust of the federal government in mental retardation, like the research thrust of NARC itself, was secondary to the interests in the humanitarian aspects of mental retardation. Nevertheless, there was a clear and explicit intertwining of the growth of the federal government's impact in mental retardation research and the development of NARC's own program. The most single important figure in the struggle during the 1950's to procure financial support necessary for advancing the programs in mental retardation was Congressman John E. Fogarty of Rhode Island, who was in constant contact with key NARC volunteers, notably Dr. Elizabeth Boggs—a chemist who developed an indefatigable interest in the mental retardation advocacy movement after the discovery, in the late 1940's, that her son was mentally retarded. Under Congressman Fogarty's energetic leadership, funds were earmarked for mental retardation in general and for mental retardation research specifically. In fiscal year 1956, $500,000 in the National Institute on Neurological Diseases and Blindness and $250,000 in the National Institute of Mental Health were set aside for mental retardation research (18).

During the late fifties a major project was in the offing—the collaborative perinatal project—which was to involve some 14 collaborating medical centers in various parts of the country to study 58,000 pregnant women during their pre- and post-natal conditions, and to study the circumstances affecting them and their children from early pregnancy until the time the child reached the age of seven years. Dr. Powers and also Dr. Glidden Brooks from the United Cerebral Palsy Associations were most active in promoting the project, which was directed by none other than Dr. Richard Masland (19).

THE KENNEDY CATALYST

One of the more significant events in the recent history of research on mental retardation was the election of John F. Kennedy as President of the United States in 1960. While he had shown no unusual interest in legislation affecting mentally retarded persons while he was in Congress, he was immediately identified with the cause when he became President. One of his first major moves—one that was to have significant consequences in the field of mental retardation—was the establishment of the National Institute of Child Health and Human Development (NICHD) as one of the National Institutes of Health. This institute gave research on child development, including research on mental retardation, a new emphasis. Dr. Robert E. Cooke, Professor of Pediatrics at Johns Hopkins and the father of two retarded children, was especially able and influential on the task force that proposed the establishment of NICHD. Dr. Cooke had long been identified with the NARC Research Program, having been its first grantee (20). This Institute was to become the monitor of the Mental Retardation Research Centers that were to be authorized by the Kennedy legislation of 1963.

Shortly after Kennedy became President, it became clear that his sister, Eunice Kennedy Shriver, would be the member of the Kennedy team most centrally involved in considering the nation's responsibilities in research, training, and service related to the prevention and management of mental retardation. She was the Kennedy's major liaison with the 27-member President's Panel on Mental Retardation established in 1961. When this prestigious group met at the White House in October of 1961, President Kennedy addressed them with these significant words, "The manner in which our nation cares for its citizens and conserves its manpower resources is more than an index to its concern for the less fortunate. It is a key to its future. Both wisdom and humanity dictate a deep interest in the physically handicapped, the mentally ill and the mentally retarded. Yet, although we have made considerable progress in the treatment of physical handicaps, although we have attacked on a broad front the problems of mental illness, although we have made great strides in the battle against disease, we as a nation have for too long postponed an intensive search for solutions to the problems of the mentally retarded. That failure should be corrected" (21).

One year later this Panel submitted its report to the President. Especially useful was a chart book to dramatize its findings (22). This Report was to have a profound effect on advancing the welfare of our mentally retarded citizens.

Many people would argue that the climax of the research effort on behalf of mentally retarded children and adults came with the legislation of 1963 which authorized the Mental Retardation Research Centers and the University Affiliated Centers for research and treatment on mental retardation and related aspects of human development. It is significant that the Joseph P. Kennedy, Jr. Foundation was instrumental in accelerating the implementation of both of these pieces of legislation by outlaying millions of dollars as matching money for the federal funds. Thus it is that many of these research centers bear the name of Kennedy in one form or another (23).

One indicator of the dramatic growth of research for the benefit of mentally retarded persons is the amount of money that has been budgeted for this purpose by the federal government. In 1950, when NARC began, no money was budgeted for mental retardation research, although perhaps as much as $200,000 from the budgets of NIMH and NINDB were used to support such research projects (24). The breakthrough came in fiscal year 1956 when, as stated above, $750,000 were specifically earmarked for mental retardation research (18). The growth from that point was phenomenal, rising to a current annual HEW mental retardation research budget of more than $31,000,000 (25). In addition, the federal government has spent $26,000,000 (matched by $17,500,000 from nonfederal sources) for the 12 mental retardation research centers and more than $41,500,000 for the 19 university affiliated centers (matched by more than $23,000,000 in nonfederal money) (23). The Congress of the United States has truly put its money "on the line" for mental retardation research!

NARC'S RESEARCH PARTICIPATION

By 1966, Dr. Abner Wolf, who replaced Dr. Powers as Chairman of the Research Advisory Board in 1961, was able to reflect on the accomplishments of the NARC Research Program (26). He noted that: 1) NARC had responded immediately to discovery of the chromosomal anomaly associated with Down's Syndrome by sponsoring a conference in 1959 on the "Etiology of Mongolism." A report of this conference was published. Dr. Josef Warkany, who has contributed a chapter to this volume on Down's Syndrome, was a principal participant. 2) NARC had participated in the support of Dr. Robert Guthrie in his development of the diagnostic screening test for PKU—which permits early dietary treatment of this inborn error of metabolism. 3) NARC had supported several projects to identify more effective ways to prevent brain damage during the birth process. 4) NARC was supporting several promising studies to counteract the effects of cultural and environmental deprivation which result in mental retardation.

OBSOLESCENCE AND REDIRECTION

However, in the four years that followed 1966, a number of factors combined to bring the NARC leadership to a position of genuine concern about the direction, and especially the impact, of the NARC research program.

Membership asked: "Why do we never hear about the results from NARC Research Projects?" "How does the NARC research effort affect the daily lives of mentally retarded children and adults?" "Why must NARC depend upon the special interest of the applicant for its research topics?" "Shouldn't NARC take an active posture in identifying the research needs of mentally retarded citizens?"

These questions arose from a number of causes. First, while the strategy of long-term support for promising young scientists was a wise one at the outset in that it encouraged an investigator to make a career commitment to mental retardation research, it had outlived its usefulness as a funding strategy. The many mental retardation research training programs and the huge federal outlay for mental retardation research had made it no longer crucial for NARC to stimulate the young investigator. Second, there was not present a viable mechanism for ongoing reporting to the NARC constituency of the results of the research that it had sponsored. Indeed, some of the research projects were so specialized as to be meaningless to their sponsors. The NARC program had either to resell the constituency on the rationale for conducting basic research, or to commit itself to a program of mission-oriented research that the constituency could understand and apply. Third, the NARC research program, which began in a position of leadership in mental retardation research, had surrendered that position and was now following in the wake of the federal programs. It seemed that there was no place for a NARC research program unless it was on the frontier of the concerns of the NARC membership.

Because of these concerns, Frank White, then President of the Association, called a moratorium on all research funding in November of 1970 and asked the senior author of this appendix, as NARC Board Coordinator for Program Services, to study the feasibility of redirecting NARC's research efforts.

My report stressed the fact that numerous federal and foundation resources had redirected their efforts toward many of the same research goals that NARC had pursued in the past (27, 28). I pointed out that NARC's efforts had played no small part in bringing about this redirection, but suggested that NARC would do well to avoid competing with programs whose resources were many times greater than its own. I suggested that NARC could better serve in the role of stimulating innovative research and research applications that would make an immediate difference in the lives of mentally retarded children and adults. This role would take maximum advantage of the Association's assets as an organization with well-defined goals and a national visibility. I saw in NARC a rare opportunity to develop a nationwide organ for the generation, the dissemination, and the implementation of research findings for the benefit of the mentally retarded.

IMPLEMENTING THE NEW RESEARCH PROGRAM

Following these recommendations, the Research Advisory Board was replaced by a Research Advisory Committee, a committee of parent as well as professional volunteers. A survey of the membership's research priorities was made through the Association's Newspaper, *Mental Retardation News* (29). From the information provided by the membership and the recommendations of the Research Advisory Committee, the NARC Board of Directors established the following five areas of research priorities (30):

Home Training Techniques
Residential Model Evaluation
Preventive Biomedical Research
Preventive Behavioral Research
Organizational Dynamics Analysis

Responsibility for developing and monitoring projects in each of these areas was assigned to specific task forces of the Research Advisory Committee. The following is a synopsis of their reports.

1. *Development and Evaluation of Techniques by Which Parents Can Train their Mentally Retarded Children at Home.*

This *Home Training* task force report by Sidney Bijou recommended that NARC focus its research in that area on the study of delivery systems that will make current materials available to mentally retarded children. Dr. Bijou felt that since adequate materials in the training area were already available, development of additional materials would be a needless duplication—that the need here was for a workable delivery system.

2. *Development and Evaluation of Alternative Models for Residential Care*

Mr. David Sokoloff is chairman of this task force. We have heard a lot of talk about the changing role of the institution, but we are sadly lacking the data that are necessary to make these changes intelligently. For example, how can we prepare institution-reared children for community residence? How do we best teach retarded adolescents the homemaking and self-care skills that are required by a normalized group home? Should group homes be composed of homogeneous or heterogeneous ages, sexes and disabilities? These are all questions about which we are desperately in need of data.

3. *Biomedical Research to Prevent Mental Retardation*

We all know that our primary target is the elimination of preventable mental retardation. According to Dr. George Jervis, chairman of this task force, we know the cause of subnormal intelligence in only about 25 percent of the cases. We need to know more about causes, and procedures for eliminating them. Furthermore, we must continue to influence preventive practices by making the advances of research publicly available.

4. *Behavioral and Environmental Research to Prevent Mental Retardation.*

During the past decade we have been increasingly aware of environmental factors that may cause mental retardation. Dr. Henry Cobb, chairman of this task force, has stressed the need for a thorough professional review of the current status of research in this area. Why do the poor have more mentally retarded children than the wealthy? How can we prevent the progressive retardation that is often associated with prolonged institutionalization?

5. *Research on the Organizational Dynamics of Volunteer Associations, Especially NARC.*

Associations, like individuals, change with age. However, unlike individuals, associations can have perpetual renewal. Dr. Wolf Wolfensberger, task force chairman in this area, emphasized that many questions must be answered to find out how! What organizational structure promotes the most effective action? What are the factors that keep an association and its units vigorous and growing?

It must be stressed that the Association has not abandoned preventive research. However, in the NARC's redirected program, the preventive priorities will be focused onto research that promises to have immediate practical impact (31). Furthermore, our board-adopted policy includes the advocacy of all research—basic and applied, medical and behavioral, operational and theoretical—that bears on the prevention or amelioration of mental retardation.

In short, the NARC Research Program promises to promote a balanced portfolio of research to benefit the daily lives of our children and to prevent mental retardation in the children of the future.

MAXIMIZING NARC'S RESEARCH IMPACT

In order to utilize fully both its tangible and intangible resources, the Research Advisory Committee has adopted three mechanisms for developing research projects in these priority areas (30). A Research Director has been employed to implement the redirected program using these mechanisms.

NARC Proposals

This is a method of initiating research projects by having NARC staff apply for foundation and federal support of specific projects—then engage the appropriate scientists to actually conduct the research. This approach assures that the association is actively involved in its research projects at every stage.

Solicited Proposals

In each of the priority areas, the Research Advisory Committee develops specific research projects. For each project, the research director prepares a prospectus for circulation to the nation's leading scientists in applied mental retardation research. This prospectus invites the submission of proposals to pursue the research in question, and fully utilizes the universities and other centers of learning in our country.

Unsolicited Proposals

In order to assure that NARC is not limited to the collective creativity of the Research Advisory Committee and its research staff, the Association reviews and supports unsolicited research proposals. Proposals for projects must lie within the priority areas and must promise immediate impact on the daily lives of mentally retarded children and adults. These proposals are initially submitted to the NARC Director of Research, closely reviewed, and then sent to the appropriate Task Force members of the Research Advisory Committee.

Whenever possible, private foundation and federal support is being sought for the bulk of the funding of all proposals, so that NARC can have maximum impact per dollar of support.

PROGRESS REPORT ON ACTIVITIES UNDER THE REDIRECTION

Now, how is the redirected program working? I can only report that all current indications are good.

The news article on the redirected program, mentioned above, reported that we have received more than 60 applications for research funding (1). To date we have funded a number of these, including the following.

Early Childhood Intervention Workshop

In the priority area of *home training* a grant has been made to Mr. David Shearer of the Portage Project in Portage, Wisconsin, to present a workshop and develop a package to describe the model and results of his very successful home training research and development project. Funded by the State of Wisconsin Department of Public Instruction, the project features a home training program in which preschool, handicapped children have made documented gains in cognitive, motoric and social skills that exceed expectations based on their previous development. Parents are taught to help their children achieve from one to five new behavior goals each week. During the week the parents keep simple but complete charts on their children's performance for each of these goals. The project is economically feasible, the cost per child being about $800 per school year. This workshop was held in Dallas, Texas, on August 9, 1973. The workshop package that results from the project will soon be available to all local Associations for Retarded Citizens.

An Analysis of the Organization Dynamics of NARC

In the priority area of *organizational dynamics* a project has been funded internally for the NARC research staff to develop a system for analyzing and interpreting data about the Association itself. The project will develop data banks based on information that is sent routinely to the NARC office and will do research projects on such topics as ARC effectiveness, membership acquisition and funding strategies. Dr. Ronald Neman is the project director.

Case Studies of Successful Community Residential Facilities

In the *residential models* priority area the Research Advisory Committee has contracted with Mr. Kurt Wehbring of San Francisco to undertake six intensive case studies of successful community residential facilities. These reports should provide valuable models for the deinstitutionalization process. Mr. Wehbring is selecting his homes in consultation with representatives of NARC, Dr. Gail O'Connor (Research Director of the Rehabilitation Research and Training Center at the University of Oregon) and Mr. Dennis Schulman of the Park Project at Harvard University.

Project to Enhance Estetrol Monitoring

It appears that levels of estetrol (an estrogen hormone) during pregnancy reflect the status of the unborn baby's sensitivity to a variety of toxic conditions. However, these levels have been very difficult to monitor in the past. Dr. Ajay Bhatnagar of the Medical College of Virginia has proposed a project to develop estetrol-specific antibody which can be easily detected in the mother's urine. This project is in the research program's *preventive biomedical* priority area.

LOOKING AHEAD: NARC'S BALANCED PORTFOLIO OF RESEARCH, RESEARCH DISSEMINATION, AND RESEARCH ADVOCACY

The essence of NARC's research posture can be summarized as follows. NARC recognizes the necessity for continuing programs of research, both "basic" and "applied," in the field of mental retardation. Basic research *is necessary* because we do not understand the fundamental mechanisms that produce large individual differences in intellectual development and in the efficiency of learning.

Continuing *basic research* is essential in such areas as genetics, biochemistry, cell physiology, metabolism, developmental psychology, learning, motivation, sensory and perceptual processes, and brain-behavior relationships. Understanding of such basic systems is necessary before one can truly understand developmental deviation that may relate to them. On the other hand, the direct study of mental retardation can lead not only to better understanding of this condition but frequently also to more general understanding of development that can be applied across the field of human development.

Applied research is necessary because there is an accumulation of basic knowledge whose application to the development of retarded persons has not yet been carefully specified. Technologies must be developed, evaluated, revised, and disseminated that will make use of existing knowledge toward improving the quality of life for retarded citizens. Untested methods abound for the care, treatment, education, and habilitation of retarded persons. Consumers of such services are not always equipped to distinguish between proven and untested methods. Given limited resources, it is most efficient to insist upon small-scale testing of service systems before implementing such strategies widely.

The members of NARC are mostly persons who have daily concern for the care, treatment, education, and habilitation of retarded children and adults. NARC has limited financial resources for its ongoing research efforts. In its first two decades (1950-1970), through its dedicated efforts to initiate general research interest in the field of mental retardation via its "Pennies for Research" financial and public informational efforts, the thrust of these efforts provided the impetus for the establishment of a national network of research and living centers in mental retardation. For these reasons, NARC has now focused its primary emphasis on applied research with respect to the direct use of its own limited funds. At the same time, an appropriate distribution of responsibility would require that other agencies, such as federal and state governments and private foundations, should more energetically assume and extend their current and future responsibility for the support of basic research in human development.

NARC will use the major portion of its research budget to support applied research, program development, program evaluation, and dissemination. Simultaneously, NARC urges its members and friends to insist upon the support by the state and federal governments of basic research in mental retardation and related aspects of human development.

NARC SUPPORTED DOWN'S SYNDROME RESEARCH

To what extent has NARC research been devoted to studies of Down's Syndrome? In order to answer the question, it is necessary to again briefly highlight some historical aspects of the NARC research program.

As previously noted, when the NARC Scientific Research Advisory Board was established in 1954, there was a dearth of research in any area of mental retardation. Accordingly, our first efforts were to learn just what was known about mental retardation and to stimulate further general interest in the area among various scientific disciplines. Such a broad focus was consistent with NARC's aim to assist *all* mentally retarded persons. However, early in the development of the research program, two biomedical areas became apparent "favorites" for research support—genetic and metabolic disorders associated with mental retardation. Between the years 1958, when NARC's review of all previous mental retardation research was published in the book *Mental Subnormality,* and 1970, when NARC undertook to redirect its research thrusts, nearly $1.5 million were expended. Of that amount, nearly $1 million were devoted to supporting genetic and metabolic research.

In 1960, Dr. Josef Warkany published, in the *Journal of Pediatrics,* a paper entitled "Etiology of Mongolism," which was a detailed report on the first national conference in which the known facts and theories concerning the etiology of Down's Syndrome were reviewed and future research was considered. The NARC Scientific Research Advisory Board sponsored this Conference. The Conference was held on October 19, 1959. The research fallout from the Conference is, of course, immeasurable. Nevertheless, that national scientific focus was brought for the first time specifically to Down's Syndrome gives evidence of NARC's commitment to Down's Syndrome research. Dr. Warkany's concluding coment, "The discovery of an extra chromosome in the cells of mongols will completely change the direction of etiological research in this area," no doubt reflected the philosophy which led NARC to devote nearly $1 million toward genetic and metabolic research.

During the 1960's, NARC supported at least six researchers whose investigations were directly or indirectly related to Down's Syndrome. A brief review of these research efforts is in order: 1) Dr. Harold O. Goodman published 11 research articles dealing with Down's Syndrome which directly or indirectly received encouragement from the NARC grant to him. His studies focused on the trisomic chromosome associated with Down's Syndrome and correlated features in blood groupings, biochemical metabolites and distinguishing morphology. 2) Dr. Gilbert Solitare's NARC supported studies investigated age-related changes in brain morphology in persons with Down's Syndrome. Dr. Solitare reported that associated with Down's Syndrome were certain specific changes not found in non-Down's Syndrome mentally retarded adults. 3) An NARC grant to Dr. Irving Wolman permitted studies of blood structure differences among Down's Syndrome and "organic" causes of mental retardation.

In addition to the 1959 conference and the three projects cited above, NARC funded three additional studies which had close relationships to ongoing Down's Syndrome research. These are: 1) One of the pioneering efforts to develop a genetic counseling service was stimulated by the NARC Grover F. Power Award granted to Dr. Harry Gordon in 1964. 2) A grant to Robert S. Tacker permitted investigation into the relationship between the age of the ovum when it is fertilized and postnatal development. These studies were related to others specifically dealing with Down's Syndrome, such as those conducted by Dr. James German (e.g., "Mongolism, Delayed Fertilization, and Human Sexual Behavior"). 3) And finally, a grant to

Dr. W. Roy Breg provided laboratory equipment for some early studies of chromosomal changes during cellular growth and division (mitosis) phases. The emphasis of this research was human chromosomal abnormalities.

In addition to the 1959 conference and the specific studies cited above, NARC played a prominent role in bringing about the landmark legislation which authorized the establishment of Mental Retardation Research Centers and University Affiliated Facilities for mental retardation research and training activities throughout our country. Since Down's Syndrome is one of the areas under exploration and investigation in these facilities, NARC must in part be credited in an indirect way for the federally sponsored research in Down's Syndrome.

It should be noted that, in accord with the Resolution of the First International Down's Syndrome Meeting to the National Association for Retarded Citizens passed at the twenty-third National Convention in Anaheim, Dr. Richard Koch, Conference Chairman of the Down's Syndrome Congress, has been asked to serve on NARC's Research Advisory Committee. Much of the impetus behind the resolution came about through NARC's co-sponsorship of this Conference. Dr. Koch's appointment to the Research Advisory Committee should further ensure that Down's Syndrome will remain a vital focus of NARC research!

With regard to future possibilities, it is clearly the case that the very limited funds which are currently available to NARC for research are insufficient to underwrite expensive biomedical research programs in Down's Syndrome or any other area. Thus, the core support for research into the molecular biology and causation of extra-chromosomal features found in Down's Syndrome must continue to come from the federal government and private foundations. On the other hand, NARC may be able to obtain research funds for less expensive studies of treatment methods for Down's Syndrome. Such research is consistent with the research redirection which has been described. NARC is able to undertake research in highly controversial areas where other organizations and foundations may not be so inclined. For example, among our constituency, there is considerable interest in and enthusiasm for the work of Dr. Mary Coleman (B-6, 5-hydroxytryptophan), Dr. Turkel (U-49 series), and Dr. Jacobs (DMSO) and other speculative treatment modalities.

Finally, representatives of the Down's Syndrome Congress may wish to formulate specific research proposals that the NARC Research Advisory Committee could seek to implement with the aid of outside funds. The alternatives for immediately beneficial research could also be selected as a discussion or workshop topic at next year's Down's Syndrome Congress Convention, wherein specific proposals could be developed and funded with NARC assistance.

SUMMARY

Looking back over the past 24 years, NARC can be proud of the contribution it has made to the growth of knowledge about mental retardation. But we are not resting. Much more needs to be done to make the results of research operational for the benefit of our mentally retarded citizens. We of the National Association for Retarded Citizens are committed to develop and maintain a posture of leadership in the support, conduct, dissemination and advocacy of research on the prevention and amelioration of mental retardation in the decades ahead.

REFERENCES

1. Redirected Research Program Underway. *Mental Retardation News.* Arlington, Texas: NARC, September, 1973, p. 2.
2. BOGGS, ELIZABETH M.: Federal legislation 1955-1965. In Wortis, Joseph (Ed.) *Mental Retardation: An Annual Review,* III New York: Grune & Stratton, 1971, p. 104.
3. *Ibid.,* p. 105.
4. *Ibid.,* p. 104.
5. Minutes from the first annual convention of the National Association for Retarded Children, Chicago, Illinois. Arlington, Texas: NARC, September 29, 1950, p. 6.
6. Minutes from the third annual convention of the National Association for Retarded Children, Chicago, Illinois. Arlington, Texas: NARC, October 12, 1952, p. 27-28.
7. Mongolism Subject of N.Y. Institute. *Children Limited,* Arlington, Texas: NARC, May-June, 1953, p. 13.
8. *Ibid.,* p. 13.
9. 21 Scientists, Educators Join NARC Research Advisory Board. *Children Limited,* Arlington, Texas: NARC, December, 1954, p. 2.

10. NARC Research Director Named. *Ibid.*, p. 2.
11. MASLAND, R. L., SARASON, S. B., and GLADWIN, T.: *Mental Subnormality.* New York: Basic Books, 1958.
12. MASLAND, R. L.: Research Survey Report, *Children Limited,* Arlington, Texas: NARC, February, 1958, p. 4.
13. SARASON, S. B. and GLADWIN, T.: The Psychological Problem. *Children Limited,* Arlington, Texas: NARC, February, 1958, p. 5.
14. Dr. Powers Lists Key Areas for NARC-Backed Research, *Children Limited,* Arlington, Texas: NARC, February, 1958, p. 6.
15. *Ibid.*, p. 6.
16. $122,880 U.S. Aid to Spur Research, *Children Limited,* Arlington, Texas: NARC, June-July, 1954.
17. BOGGS, *op. cit.*, p. 108-111.
18. $750,000 Grant OK'd in Congress, *Children Limited,* Arlington, Texas: NARC, March, 1955, p. 1.
19. BOGGS, *op. cit.*, p. 107.
20. NARC Starts Active Support of Research Work, *Children Limited,* Arlington, Texas: NARC, July, 1958, p. 6.
21. KENNEDY, J. F.: A national plan to combat mental retardation: A statement by the president regarding the need for a national plan in mental retardation, Washington: U.S. Government Printing Office, 1962.
22. President's Panel on Mental Retardation. *Chart Book: Mental Retardation.* Washington: U.S. Government Printing Office, 1963.
23. (HEW) Secretary's Committee on Mental Retardation. *Mental Retardation Construction Program.* Washington: U.S. Government Printing Office, 1971.
24. BOGGS, *op. cit.*, p. 105.
25. CONLEY, R. W.: *The Economics of Mental Retardation.* Baltimore: Johns Hopkins Press, 1973, p. 140-142.
26. WOLF, A. NARC Supports Many Important Research Projects. *Children Limited,* Arlington, Texas: NARC, August-September, 1966, p. 6.
27. MENOLASCINO, F. J.: Future Course of Research Efforts of the National Association for Retarded Children: A Recommendation. DR #8485. Arlington, Texas: NARC, April 22, 1971.
28. The NARC Research Program: A New Direction. *Action Together,* Arlington, Texas: NARC, August, 1971.
29. NARC Research Program Requests Your Participation. *Mental Retardation News,* Arlington, Texas: NARC, October, 1971, p. 8.
30. The NARC Research Program: A Report on New Directions, *Action Together,* Arlington, Texas: NARC, January, 1973.
31. Research Policy Statement: National Association for Retarded Children. DR #992, Arlington, Texas: NARC, July 21, 1973.

Index